Interprofessional issues in community
and primary health care

Also by Patricia Owens

COMMUNITY CARE AND SEVERE PHYSICAL DISABILITY
NURSING IN CONFLICT (*with Howard Glennerster*)

Also by John Carrier

MEDICAL NEGLIGENCE: Complaints and Compensation
(*with Ian Kendall*)
SOCIALISM AND THE NHS (*edited with Ian Kendall*)

Also by John Horder

THE FUTURE GENERAL PRACTITIONER : Learning and Teaching
THE WRITINGS OF JOHN HUNT

Interprofessional issues in community and primary health care

Edited by

Patricia Owens

John Carrier

and

John Horder

MACMILLAN

First published 1995 by
MACMILLAN PRESS LTD
Houndmills, Basingstoke, Hampshire RG21 2XS
and London
Companies and representatives
throughout the world

ISBN 0–333–59565–3

A catalogue record for this book is available
from the British Library.

10 9 8 7 6 5 4 3 2
04 03 02 01 00 99 98 97 97

Printed in Great Britain by
Antony Rowe Ltd, Chippenham, Wiltshire.

Contents

The contributors   vii

Preface   xi
John Horder

Introduction   1
Patricia Owens and John Carrier

Section One: Theoretical contexts

1   Professionalism and interprofessionalism in health
and community care: some theoretical issues   9
John Carrier and Ian Kendall

2   Professionals and management   37
Patricia Owens and Heather Petch

3   Ethical and resource issues in health and social care   57
Andrew Wall

4   The market and professional frameworks   71
Anna Cohen

Section Two: Interprofessional collaboration in action

5   Elderly care   95
Gail Wilson and Julie Dockrell

6   Child protection   111
Elizabeth Birchall

7   Mental health services   137
Roslyn Corney

8   Palliative care   165
Patricia Owens

9   Primary health care   185
Margot Jefferys

Section Three: Inside teamwork

10 Learning to work effectively in teams   205
      Peter Pritchard

Index   233

The contributors

Elizabeth Birchall has worked for many years in various Social Services Departments at field and managerial level. From 1987 to 1992 she worked with Christine Hallett at the University of Stirling on a major project investigating interprofessional co-ordination in child protection work. Her most recent publication is 'The frequency of child abuse – what do we really know?', in O. Stevenson (ed.), *Child Abuse: Public Policy and Professional Practice* (Harvester Wheatsheaf, 1989).

John Carrier is a Senior Lecturer in Social Policy at the London School of Economics, and has been in higher education for over twenty years. His research interests are in social policy and the law and health services. He is Vice-Chairman of the Royal Free Hospital Trust and CAIPE. He has collaborated with Ian Kendall on a number of publications, of which their most recent is *Medical Negligence: Complaints and Compensation* (Avebury Press, 1990).

Anna Cohen is a social anthropologist who has worked in psychiatric hospitals in Italy and on rural development and health care in India. More recently she has carried out a project on the introduction of the internal market in the NHS and the contrasting models of health care held by clinicians and managers.

Roslyn Corney is Professor of Psychology at the University of Greenwich. Her main research interests are the evaluation of counselling and psychotherapy, investigating changes due to GP fundholding, and examining the roles of attached and employed mental health professionals in general practice. She is the editor of *Developing Communication and Counselling Skills in Medicine* and *Counselling in General Practice*, published by Routledge & Kegan Paul.

John Horder was President of the Royal College of General Practitioners from 1979 to 1982, and a GP in London for many years in a

Health Centre. He has been Chairman of the Centre for the Advancement of Interprofessional Education in Primary Health and Community Care since 1987.

Margot Jefferys was Professor of Medical Sociology at Bedford College, London University, until her retirement in 1982. She is currently Visiting Professor in the Centre of Medical Law and Ethics at King's College, London. She has written many articles on British health and welfare services. In 1983 she published *Re-thinking General Practice* with Hessie Sachs (Tavistock Publications).

Ian Kendall is Associate Dean at the University of Portsmouth and has been deeply involved for many years in nursing and social work education. He is Co-author with John Carrier of *Health and the National Health Service*, published by Athlone Press.

Patricia Owens has worked in the NHS and Social Services, and trained as a social anthropologist at Cambridge University. She was Director of CAIPE at the London School of Economics from 1991 to 1993. Her most recent publications are *Nursing in Conflict*, with Howard Glennerster (Macmillan, 1990), and *Implementing Fundholding in General Practice*, with Howard Glennerster and Manos Matsaganis (Open University Press, 1994).

Heather Petch currently works for CHAR, an organisation which promotes better services for homeless people. She has a particular interest in health and homelessness, and is the author of two reports on special health and social services in inner London for homeless people.

Peter Pritchard, who was a general practitioner in Oxfordshire, has worked on team development for a number of years. More recently he has published, with his son James Pritchard, a management consultant in industry, a workbook entitled *Developing Teamwork in Primary Health Care* (Oxford University Press, 1992).

Andrew Wall is a Senior Fellow in the Health Services Management Centre, University of Birmingham. He was a Chief Executive, and worked in the National Health Services for twenty years. His most recent publications are *Ethics and the Health Service Manager*

(King's Fund Institute, 1989), *The Reorganised National Health Service* (with Ruth Levitt, 4th edn, revised 1993) and *Values in the NHS* (Institute of Health Service Managers, 1993).

Preface

This book stems from close collaboration between the National Centre for the Advancement of Interprofessional Education (CAIPE) and the London School of Economics, during a period when the centre enjoyed the hospitality of the School's Department of Social Science and Administration. It starts from two beliefs – first that collaboration in health and social care benefits patients and clients, who are likely to suffer when it is absent; second, that shared learning can be a valuable way of improving collaboration.

Neither of these beliefs is new, but before the centre was planned in 1984, there was no continuing, independent organisation at national level which made them its main concern. There were, however, many places in this country where learning was sometimes shared between more than one profession, as the Centre's 1988 national survey later showed. Since that time, several other organisations have also started at national level, with aims which overlap, but are not identical. Meanwhile, changes resulting from the Children Act 1989 and the NHS and Community Care Act 1990, together with the world-wide problem of rising health-care costs, have made the need for collaboration between professions yet more necessary, and have called existing professional tasks and boundaries into question. A response from educationists to these changes is essential. Uniprofessional responses are not sufficient or appropriate. In the Introduction we identify the groups in the population for which collaborative care is especially important.

This Centre aims to promote shared learning and to support the many people who are offering it in the UK. It collects and disseminates relevant information, puts people and organisations in touch with one another, organises national conferences, publishes a twice-yearly bulletin and has commissioned and carried out a number of research projects. It has from the start included among its trustees and council members social workers, doctors, nurses, professions allied to medicine, managers and educationists. Membership of the centre is open to all who are concerned to promote collaborative

xi

practice through shared learning. This book focuses on the major issues which confront health and social care professionals learning and working together in our services today.

JOHN HORDER
Chairman, CAIPE, 1994

Introduction

This book explores the issues that surround interprofessional education in health and community care. The idea that different professionals need to work together to provide better services for people is not simply accepted, but analysed in a variety of theoretical and practical frameworks. The contributors to this book have addressed the issues that surround interprofessional working in the contexts of the historical development of services, organisational theory, ethical frameworks, the perspective of group dynamics and the economic background against which debates about the future of professional and interprofessional work and education have taken place. These core themes are carried through and analysed more specifically in relation to community services, mental health services, child protection, continuing care, the care of the elderly and primary health care.

The aim is to provide a text which will contribute to the knowledge and understanding of interprofessional relationships and can be used as a basic guide to the issues involved. These issues will be with us for decades to come, even if the legislation and economic framework changes. Dramatic changes in the 1980s in the NHS and other public welfare service systems have highlighted the increasing need for close co-operation between professional groups. But differences in educational backgrounds, financial structures, expectations, roles and systems create barriers to mutual understanding. The major change in the NHS since the early 1980s has been the introduction of general management, and in the 1990s, the purchaser – provider split.

With the resulting change from all-providing DHAs to Trusts, health care professionals have been drawn into fields much wider than their purely professional concerns, such as budgeting, allocation and distribution of scarce resources. These changes create demands for new approaches to be adopted for education so that improved collaboration can take place. Professionals need to assume not just shared goals, but also shared meanings about priorities, good practice, and quality assurance. In the important areas such as care of elderly or disabled people, child protection and health promotion, the teamwork approach is essential to providing effective, efficient and responsive services for patients and clients. Changing demands have forced purchasers and providers to think in terms of service specifications, and these are dependant on training and re-training, and education and re-education. The process is continuous.

In Europe, the changing face of health care in developed industrial societies presents challenges to the future education and training of health care professionals to meet new needs. The impact of demographic transformations and economic constraints presents different ethical problems concerning the equitable distribution of resources. Changing ideologies of health care suggest to the World Health Organization and others a need for a fundamental reassessment of training and education in the field of health care (WHO, 1991), particularly in the area of medical education.

The unifying theme of this book is that the development of better community-based services depends to a large extent on a multidisciplinary approach to health care. However, the composition and skill-mix in services in determined in many cases by traditional assumptions concerning needs, or the particular contributions of different professionals. Change is, therefore, required but altering roles or boundaries is not easy to achieve without a slow and sensitive process of re-education. Such a process focuses sharply the education and training issues which all professional will have to address in the future. If old boundaries disappear, where is the fixed mark of the professional claim to be located? The answer will be in the absolutes of standards, not the relativities of the shifting political objectives.

Questions are, therefore, raised about professional integrity, the quality of professional training, the maintenance of standards, and flexibility of service delivery. These are very complex. The challenges of the 1990s in health and social care require us to re-examine the relationship of professionals within the major organisations delivering health and social care services. We also need to have a greater understanding of the dynamics of the relationships between different professional groups, and the processes involved in working across the structural boundaries of various service areas. This need is now being recognised by health authorities, and the professional bodies responsible for training; it is central to the future of such services.

The first four chapters of this book set the scene of interprofessional work, and examine the *theoretical issues*. In Chapter 1, Carrier and Kendall analyse the hypothesis that interprofessional collaboration is a prerequisite for an efficient and effective delivery of health and social care. They focus the issues of power, prestige and rivalry, hierarchy and bureaucracy which characterise professional work within our welfare systems. These themes are set against the changing political and social environment of services and the greater involvement of consumers, informal carers and voluntary groups.

Owens and Petch, in Chapter 2, develop some of these themes further, especially those of professional autonomy in relation to bureaucratic structures, managerialism versus professionalism. Focusing on doctors, nurses and social workers, the impact of the recent reforms embodied in the NHS and Community Care Act 1990 is analysed, drawing upon the research of Owens, Glennerster, Matsaganis and Petch. They describe how the development of a managerial culture, the growth of a corporate ideology, and the involvement of professionals in resource allocation decisions has had the fundamental effect of dismantling traditional professional hierarchies of power.

In Chapter 3, Wall examines the complexity of pushing resource allocation decisions down to service provision level. The issue here is that the face-to-face relationship between the clinician and patient, involving the autonomy of the professional, may stimulate conflicts with the more global view of the manager. The issues of equity across services made by managers are finely balanced against the intensely individual resource allocation decisions made by doctors.

Cohen (Chapter 4) plays a different tune on the same theme when she focuses on the use of language by managers and professionals in relation to the market philosophy in health care. She describes a world where images and rhetoric are 'consciously manipulated in order to control other players', thus gaining access to power and resources. The necessity of going beyond these narrow professional concerns, and addressing the problems of individual access to the network of care, is placed in the context of the competitive forces in the health and social care market.

In the second section of the book, the first four chapters explore different facets of care in the community. Wilson and Dockrell, in Chapter 5, illustrate the complex and diverse health and social needs of elderly people. The number of professionals needed to attend to these often leaves users and carers in a state of confusion. The authors draw upon their own work with groups of professionals to explore the difficult issue of co-operative work between these individual workers. The role of the expert is seen to be both beneficial and threatening, as it leads to the creation of stereotypes and inhibits the crossing of organisational boundaries in the interests of patients and clients. The effect of economic constraints and competition may encourage interprofessional collaboration, but if professionals feel threatened, traditional divisions may be reinforced.

Birchell, in Chapter 6, draws upon her study of co-ordinated approaches to child protection, covering the relevant literature on the subject, survey data and interviews with key professionals in this field. The role of the social worker is examined in detail in the context of the widespread political pressures to promote interprofessional collaboration. She describes the difficulty in mixing therapeutic care with the social control aspect of child abuse work, and the incompatibility of some of the values and perspectives of the professionals involved. These dimensions are overlaid by differences in local policies, lack of technical consensus across professionals and inequalities in power relationships.

The necessity for interprofessional collaboration and the difficulty of achieving it are analysed by Corney in Chapter 7, in a discussion of the mental health services. She asks why we should think that interprofessional collaboration is a necessary prerequisite for better service delivery. Her chapter covers the historical background and recent legislation, and gives a wide-ranging account of the substantial literature on this subject. A major conclusion based on the author's own investigations is that the primary health care team has a key role in providing services which are accessible, non-stigmatising and give continuous long-term care. She suggests, however, that these services are also of uneven quality and spread.

Owens (Chapter 8) follows with a discussion of the role of the palliative care team. This is an area where there has been a conscious effort by the hospice movement to develop close working relationships between professionals. The discussion is prefaced by a brief account of changing attitudes to and cultural perspectives on death in Western societies over time, and the growing power of the medical profession which is associated with technical advances. The chapter concludes that society isolates death in institutions, and that professionals in all health and social care groups have, hitherto, lacked the necessary education and training to respond appropriately to public expectations.

The final chapter in this section is devoted by Jefferys to Primary Health Care (Chapter 9). The key role of the doctor is one that is central in most, if not all the previous chapters. But Jefferys, in her clear analysis of the development of primary health care teams, describes the difficult evolution of this concept, and 'the cottage industry' approach of general practitioners. The reforms since the

1960s have gradually strengthened their position and encouraged GPs to include others in their services, and collaborate with a wider variety of professionals in responding to social and psychological, as well as medical needs of patients.

Finally, Pritchard's chapter (Chapter 10) takes us inside the world of teamwork. He gives a wide-ranging, stimulating and informative account of the literature on teamwork, with a focus on the primary health care team. His special insight as a former GP gives this chapter an added edge as he speaks with the voice of experience.

He covers some of the strategies which have developed to encourage teamwork in order to achieve targets set in *Health of the Nation* (1992). The author identifies and describes different methods which should assist professionals to achieve a unity of objectives and working practices which are shared. These methods have a general application for all interprofessional groups coming together to serve a common purpose in the interests of patients or clients and their carers. Pritchard also suggests a framework for action and interprofessional education.

The common theme of all chapters is that professionals can no longer regard their work as strictly autonomous. The NHS and Community Care Act 1990 has set an agenda for action which requires joint working across agency boundaries, and as such, it has been instrumental in breaking down traditional professional barriers determining a shared approach to the provision of care. Carrier and Kendall finish their chapter with a verse about the need to keep knowledge secure and safe and not spread it about too much. However, the role of the expert is now being questioned, and the need for the sharing of expertise, the pooling of knowledge and the crossing of traditional boundaries has become, not a choice, but an essential ingredient of delivering high quality social and health care. The importance of professionals in determining the shape of services and maintaining standards is also confirmed and made clear.

The editors hope that this book will give students of interprofessional work valuable insights into both the obstructions and avenues to success in working together more effectively. It is hoped that the latter will prove in the long term to be more durable than the former.

1994   PATRICA OWENS
                                               JOHN CARRIER

SECTION ONE

Theoretical
Contexts

1 Professionalism and interprofessionalism in health and community care: some theoretical issues

John Carrier and Ian Kendall

Chapter summary

In this chapter the authors examine the concept of professionalism in the context of current changes in health and welfare services. The exclusivity and autonomous status of the professional within bureaucratic public service organisations is challenged by the concept of interprofessional collaboration, which demands that professionals share resources, knowledge and responsibility. Issues of professional and political power are analysed in relation to public policy which advocates a market in health and social care and a greater emphasis on voluntarism and consumerism. The authors suggest that these changes may lead inevitably to a process of deprofessionalisation.

Introduction

To justify an interprofessional approach to the delivery of health and social care, it is first of all necessary to be confident about the base from which professional claims to service delivery are made. The characteristic structure of welfare services in industrial societies was described many years ago as involving 'specialised bureaucratic agencies, professionally staffed' (Wilensky and Lebeaux, 1965, p. 230). This perspective has informed a substantial social science literature concerning the role of welfare professionals, the operation of welfare bureaucracies and a widely reported conflict between professional and bureaucratic modes of work.

Professionalism and bureaucracy emerge as pejorative labels from much of this social science analysis and evaluation. Indeed, the most recent health and community care policy agenda in Britain based on concepts of consumerism, purchaser–provider splits, privatisation

9

and welfare pluralism, might be assumed to have drawn heavily on this social science literature, with social scientists acting, presumably unwittingly, as 'the enemy within'. Certainly the recent policy agenda seems to reflect a deep-rooted mistrust of the sort of public service professionalism associated with 'specialised bureaucratic agencies, professionally staffed'.

In seeking to gauge the significance of the changes now being implemented, we hope to trace possible futures for multiprofessional and interprofessional work – the virtues of which were identified some time before internal markets and purchaser–provider splits entered the policy debate and the vocabulary of health and social care professionals (see, for example, National Development Group for the Mentally Handicapped, 1976, pp. 7–8). A related issue will be the extent to which the new arrangements for purchasing and providing health and social care might displace traditional forms of public service professionalism and lead to the establishment of a different characteristic structure of welfare services.

For the purposes of this chapter, we define multiprofessional work as a co-operative enterprise in which traditional forms and divisions of professional knowledge and authority are retained. More radically, interprofessional work implies a willingness to share and indeed give up exclusive claims to specialised knowledge and authority, if the needs of clients can be met more efficiently by other professional groups.

The National Health Service and Community Care Act 1990 may be regarded as either a threat or an opportunity in relation to the development of multiprofessional co-operation and interprofessional collaboration in health and social care. A range of possibilities includes, on the one hand, community nurses, occupational therapists and social workers in cut-throat competition with one another for scarce and sought-after contracts to provide services; and on the other hand, the development of new, innovative and collaborative interprofessional service providers, released from the artificial constraints of the previous budgetary and organisational divisions between health (NHS) and social care (social services departments).

The latter may sound attractive, but it is necessary to be clear about the questions that surround professional work before we can be certain that such collaborations will successfully meet both the needs of service-users and the aspirations of current and future professionals. An obvious question is whether all is well within the professional worlds of health and social care?

To this end this chapter eschews examining the detail of the current legislative and policy changes in the fields of health and social care, these being addressed in other chapters. Instead, we explore some of the theoretical debates that may inform practical attempts to make the new legislation work, and which should be considered in discussions of interprofessional activity, relations, and education. An examination of these debates necessitates a brief introduction to the established theoretical perspectives on professions and the process of professionalisation, in order to distil the key themes that emerge from the social science critiques of the professions. Following reviews of interprofessional relations and the most recent health and community care policy agenda, we conclude with an examination of alternatives to traditional forms of professionalism and the potential role of, and possible questions associated with, an interprofessional approach in health and community care.

Professions and professionalisation

Why is professional status and activity so deeply entrenched in the social structures of modern societies? One set of social science explanations has rested upon defining the professional life as being based upon the possession of certain attributes such as the work of professionals is dignified, skilled and proficient, and undertaken for remuneration, rather than voluntarily or charitably provided. These attributes bestow professional authority. Further, it is argued that the public can trust the functionally specific competence of a professional and that this is universally recognised; elevating professional neutrality above personal feelings and thus guaranteeing an orientation to the service of the client rather than to the aggrandisement of the self. Finally, professional practice is dominated by a recourse to theory when confronting client problems. This practice is based upon a long training period, giving to the professional graduate a shared community of ideas and colleagues. It is assumed that all professional training instils in the trainee a commitment to a code of ethics, which allows professional autonomy based upon trust to advise clients whose dependence upon that advice makes them vulnerable and powerless. Professional life, therefore, is above all a claim to sapiential authority, high ethical standards and autonomy based upon the judicious use of discretion and judgement on behalf of clients.

An alternative perspective locates professional activity within systems of power in which professions enjoy high status and autonomy in their working lives. The distinctive qualities of professional knowledge are functional for the professional, rather than the client and the wider community. The privileges of professional status are actively sought by occupational groups through processes of social exclusion. The resulting claims to exclusive areas of expertise and for lengthy periods of training may be presumed less likely to stand up to objective, critical scrutiny. Inequalities in professional status may be associated with the class and gender composition of the different professions, rather than their knowledge-bases and expertise. In-deed, the law and the church are hardly scientific and it has been said that their status rests more upon them being gentlemen's occu-pations than their technically exclusive skills (see, for example, Marshall, 1963). Freidson adds a persuasive economic interpretation of this status, suggesting that professions are a form of cartel having 'the exclusive right to offer specific services, a right sustained by the state . . .' (Freidson, 1986, pp. 63–4).

Thus the growth of contemporary professions has attracted a range of accounts, extending from an essentially positive perspective ident-ifying the functions and inevitability of professionalisation for indus-trial societies, to an essentially pejorative perspective identifying the process of professionalisation with social exclusion and the aggrega-tion of power and status. Following even the most cursory examin-ation of the social science literature, it is difficult to avoid the sense that the latter end of the continuum is somewhat overloaded with a range of competing and complementary (but far from complimen-tary) perspectives (P. Wilding, 1982, especially ch. 4).

Professions against the world, Part One: the theorists

> To acquire one critique may be regarded as a misfortune; to acquire a crowd of critiques looks like carelessness. (with apologies to Lady Brack-nell and Oscar Wilde)

Their critics are respecters of neither professional claims nor political boundaries. Both ends of the conventional political spectrum are well-represented. From the left, the professions are represented at best middle-class dominated and at worst an integral part of systems of class dominance and inequalities. From the right, the professions have conspired to escape the liberating forces of competitive free markets and thus sacrificed efficiency and consumer choice. These conventional political approaches occupy this seemingly overcrowded territory, with feminist perspectives citing the male dominance of the more prestigious professions and the role of these professions as part of the broader patriarchal nature of contemporary society.

Studies of the politics of welfare have for many years identified the powerful interest group role of professional groups, causing offence to various democratic principles. The role of the medical profession and the setting up of the National Health Service has served as a classic example. There seems a rather obvious link between the observation that 'the only person not represented round the Minister's table was the patient' (Willcocks, 1967, p. 33) and an outcome in which the nationalisation of the hospitals is identified with 'the aspirations of parts of the medical profession' (Abel-Smith, 1964, p. 488); the structure of the service 'owes more to the opinion of the doctors than to political and public opinion' (Titmuss, 1968, p. 235); and the doctors emerge as perhaps the major beneficiaries of the introduction of the new service (Titmuss, 1968, p. 241).

The professional interest has been characterised as operating in certain directions, most notably in terms of the maximisation of individual and group autonomy and the minimisation of lay (including democratic) control. Examples include the medical profession's opposition to local government involvement in health care (Titmuss, 1968, p. 235) and the teaching profession's opposition to parental participation in school government (Hughes *et al.*, 1980, p. 196). Indeed, the former was sufficiently successful to keep the issue off the post-war policy agenda apart from a brief, tentative appearance in the First Green Paper on NHS reorganisation in 1968 (Ministry of Health, 1968).

This exclusion of lay incursions into professional activity also serves as part of the 'technocracising of politics'. Issues are defined as being essentially technical, to be resolved by the 'professional experts', serving to limit the power and influence of both public representatives and welfare consumers. Indeed, professionals are seen as posing particular problems for notions of accountability within state welfare. Their claims to individual and group autonomy (peer review) cut across conventional lines of accountability; the latter may be difficult enough to sustain in the context of 'big government' without the added complication of a 'reliance on experts and professionalism' (Day and Klein, 1987, p. 2). Thus these occupations whose attributes demand close regulation and scrutiny on behalf of the wider public interest are not readily susceptible to such regulation and scrutiny, despite their employment status as public servants.

In addition to their general anti-democratic bias, the professions also stand accused of using their power and status to establish and maintain particular definitions of health and social needs, and particular responses to these needs. Thus the perceived biases of the NHS in favour of hospital-based intervention in episodes of acute health problems, and the relative neglect of preventive measures, may both be at least partially attributable to these forms of health care being defined as respectively 'interesting' and 'uninteresting' by a range of health professionals. That services for elderly people with chronic health problems and for people with mental health problems are justifiably labelled 'Cinderella services', is also attributed to the professional interests of a range of health and social care professions (see, for example, Royal Commission on the NHS, 1979, ch. 6).

To this catalogue of critiques we might add the views of Ward on the housing and planning professions – his criticism of the planners' 'preoccupation with their own professionalism' and his advocacy of the 'dethronement of expertise and the reliance on ordinary people's experience' (Ward, 1976, pp. 114 and p. 141); and the views of Illich on health and education professions: 'professionals . . . tell you what you need . . . they claim the powers to prescribe . . . they not only advertise what is good, but ordain what is right' (Illich, 1978, p. 49).

The health and social care professions stand accused of an unjustified mystification and monopolisation of knowledge; and the management of scarce resources via gatekeeper roles that presume they 'know what's best'. In this context of a veritable catalogue of critiques, it is not clear that professionals will wish to seek out the problematic territory of interprofessional collaboration. But of course if their lack of enchantment with such collaboration is understandable, their failure to explore its potential serves merely to add to the broader disenchantment with professionals and professionalism. This is particularly so when this failure appears as a factor in deficiencies in health and social care policies and practices which have visible, and at times tragic, consequences.

Professions against each other

Do all professions share a similar status? There has been another debate, frequently linked with those in welfare occupations, concerning the claims to this ideal type of professional status. Key health and social care professions – for example, social work and nursing – have been consigned to the category of 'semi-profession' on account of the perceived limitations of their knowledge-base, training and autonomy (Etzioni, 1969). The latter is seen as particularly constrained by a work-base in state welfare bureaucracies. Democratic accountability and bureaucratic hierarchies are presumed to imply a degree of lay interference in professional activity which is not commensurate with the traditional ideal of professionalism. Inequalities in professional status have also been linked to the concept of the 'virtuoso role' made up of a particular blend of esoteric knowledge and skills which involves a particular degree of autonomy and social distance (see, for example, Nokes, 1967). The barrister and surgeon obviously qualify for this status; the specialist social worker working with people with learning difficulties obviously may not!

The concept of a hierarchy of professions differentiated by full and semi-professional status has a particular relevance for the health and social care professions which have contrasting histories and contrasting contemporary circumstances with regard to such central professional characteristics as the length of training, the legal status of registration and the right to practise. The latter provides a clear empirical base for both lay and professional perceptions that there are significant differences in the expertise and status of, for example, doctors, nurses and social workers.

At this point we may encounter an obvious barrier to interprofessional collaboration around such issues as confidentiality. If it is presumed that the 'semi-professions' are in a number of respects – ethical codes, legal status, political power – less well-placed to respect and adhere to 'traditional professional practices', there will be an understandable reluctance to share information and work together as equal partners. This unwillingness to collaborate may be equally understandable through the model of professions as status and power-seeking occupations. If hard-fought-for professional territories (and associated statuses) are to be effectively maintained, it may seem highly inappropriate to share any territory with other professional groups – most obviously those of a perceived lower status.

Whether motivated by the service ideal or professional self-interest, it has been widely asserted that collaboration between health and social care professionals is lacking in quantitative and qualitative terms. The most graphic and tragic examples have been the series of enquiries into apparent failings of the child care services provided by local authority social services departments. From the Maria Colwell Report (1974) to the Butler- Sloss Report (1988) into the rise in the diagnosis of child sexual abuse in Cleveland, one recurring theme was that key child care professionals – doctors, nurses, social workers, teachers – did not readily share assumptions or concerns. The same could be said of lawyers and police officers.

Professionals and professionalism appear as central issues in relation to community care. Descriptions of community care services invariably include professionals (doctors, nurses, social workers) as one of their identifying features. For policies for community care there is a very lengthy history of failures to deliver the sort of professional collaboration to which service-users might feel reasonably entitled. This history is at least partially entangled in issues of professional power and the politics of policy-making, for whilst the different professional groups may have different histories, and have been associated with different professional statuses, nevertheless there are areas of similarity. Each of these groups possesses a given share of power associated with professionalism and the influence which flows from this can be demonstrated by a brief examination of post-war health and community care policies.

The apparent ability of most of the medical profession to distance themselves from local government when the NHS was established, reinforced the isolation of the solo community-based general practitioner from local authority employed community nursing colleagues in domiciliary midwifery, district nursing and health visiting. The so-called 'Doctors' Charter' of 1966, allied to other changes, including increasing government expenditure on health centre construction, encouraged at least GPs to work together in group practices. When the Health Services and Public Health Act (1968) enabled local authorities to arrange cross-boundary visiting by their community nursing staff, the health centre-based primary health care team started to become a reality.

However, by the time this long-argued for, and long-heralded concept, was being put into practice, it had already been recognised for some time that effective community care required a collaborative enterprise between not just health professionals, but between health and social care personnel. This enterprise was clearly not facilitated by the separation of personnel and services between a tripartite NHS and local government (and within local government between district and county councils – and within the councils between different departments).

The 1964–70 Labour government responded to these and other concerns, by initiating parallel restructurings of the NHS, local government and the personal social services. In 1968 the First Green Paper on NHS reorganisation indicated a solution to the administrative, budgetary and professional divisions constraining community care, by suggesting that a unified NHS might be located in a reformed local government (Ministry of Health, 1968), presumably on the unitary model advocated subsequently by the Redcliffe-Maud Royal Commission (Redcliffe-Maud, 1969).

At this point the government was made aware of the continuing distaste of the medical profession for anything resembling local government control. The Second Green Paper set the scene for a unification of health services outside of local government (DHSS, 1970). Meanwhile there was acceptance of the recommendations of the social work dominated Seebohm Committee for unifying social work and related services in a social services department (Seebohm Report, 1968). The local authority health departments, wherein some modest degree of health and social care collaboration might have been observed, disappeared in accordance with 'the professional principle' set down in the Second Green Paper (DHSS, 1970, p. 10, para. 31). All that is social work-related was to remain in local government in a new social services department; and all that was medical and nursing elated was to move outside of local government. At considerable expense, and with detailed arrangements much influenced by key professional groups, this lengthy restructuring process came to an end in 1974 with the success of policies for community care precariously dependent on the bridging of a health and social care division more clearly delineated in administrative, financial and professional terms than at any previous stage in the history of post-war health and community care policies. For the mental health services, Jones commented that the effect could be to make doctors and nurses the rulers of a 'health' empire, while social workers become the rulers of a welfare 'empire'; subsequently noting the disappearance of anything resembling active and specialised mental health services (Jones, 1972, p. 343 and Jones, 1983, pp. 218–34).

A strong lead on behalf of interprofessional working was subsequently given by the Royal Commission on the NHS in 1979. The dominant criticism by the Commission was directed at the over-elaborate system for delivering health care and the lack of true joint collaboration between professions. One of the Commission's research reports also contained a note of caution to ideas that ending administrative and financial divisions would, of itself generate the sought-after interprofessional collaboration. The assumption that institutional change will 'of itself, cause good working together of professional groups with different expertise, social values and traditions of relations with clients' they labelled the 'organisational fallacy'; the belief that 'conflicts of objectives will be resolved by bringing all together in one system' they labelled the 'unitary fallacy' (Royal Commission on the NHS, 1978, pp. 223–32).

The existing health and social care division was the subject of a series of critical reports in the 1980s from the House of Commons Social Services Committee, the Audit Commission and Sir Roy Griffiths. All commented upon the problems of the organisational and professional divisions which prevented a truly responsive and tailor-made service to well-defined client needs (Social Services Committee, 1985, para. 96; Audit Commission, 1986, p. 3; Griffiths, 1988). There appeared to be a wide-ranging consensus that the organisational arrangements which had to a degree been sought after by the health and social care professions, and the rationale for which was existing divisions between those professions, were not providing the sort of services required.

It should come as no surprise that calls for interprofessional collaboration have proved to be more an aspiration than an easily achieved reality. Such collaboration implies the sharing of knowledge; respect for individual autonomy of different professional groups and administrators; the surrender of professional territory where necessary; and a shared set of values concerning appropriate responses to shared definitions of need. Professions, whether defined in terms of either altruistic service-ideals or conspiratorial power-seeking, are likely to find this an ambitious and demanding agenda. None the less there seemed to be a *prima facie* case for a policy agenda that was less responsive to interprofessional sensitivities, and more demanding of interprofessional collaboration, if the interests of service-users were to be met.

Professions against the world, Part Two: the policy-makers

The contents of *Working for Patients* (Department of Health, 1989a) and *Caring for People* (Department of Health, 1989b) seem to indicate that the social science criticisms made of professional activity have found their way into policy papers. Both these papers suggest it as almost axiomatic that the failure of interprofessional collaboration must now be disciplined by the strengths of the market-place. As such the reports by the Audit Commission and Sir Roy Griffiths take on a new significance because they lay down standards of practice and quantifiable targets for health and social care; and furthermore they do this by suggesting that the internal market, the purchaser–provider split (in health), the new 'skill mixes', and the key-worker/care-worker will act as the medium for interprofessional working.

The problem immediately seen with such an approach is that it represents the antithesis of what professional claims for high professional practice stand for. These claims are that professional judgements about client needs are often by their very nature unquantifiable; that quantification leads to performance league tables which become the dominant measure of success, thus devaluing the content of care; and that the introduction of a cash nexus into the relationship between the purchaser and provider can lead to a slippery slope in which professional judgements are 'bought and negotiated' rather than accepted as of right.

In this context, it is not surprising that four concerns are to be found voiced in one way or another throughout the health and social care professions. These are that markets, or quasi-markets, inevitably lead to deprofessionalisation and thus the commodification of service; that there is an inevitable de-skilling when cheaper services are sought (this especially so with regard to the use of care assistants and support workers); that dilution of standards and quality becomes inevitable; and that the decentralisation of decision-making leads to a loss of a co-ordinating standard-setting culture.

These changes in the major health and social care services, and the implications and criticisms suggested above, appear to provide an unhelpful and almost disabling context in which to discuss interprofessional collaboration. Indeed, the critics of the current policy agenda may be more inclined to see it as a precursor of the end of professionalism rather than the herald of a brave new dawn of interprofessional working!

The world without professions

What does professionalism in health and social care involve? One significant strand is that key decisions on the allocation of and access to resources are based on, or even controlled by, professional discretion derived from knowledge and expertise. This mode of decision-making we might characterise as individualised professional discretion.

Given the array of critiques directed at the professions, one is inevitably led to ask whether indeed the world would be a better place without the professions? Given the most recent policy agenda one is also led to ask whether it is the intention of the government to dispense with the professions – or at least to diminish significantly their role in some areas of health and community care.

The alternatives in theory

It is certainly possibly to identify alternatives to individualised professional discretion in health and welfare, the most obvious of which, embodied in our opening definition of the key characteristics of health and welfare agencies, is a *bureaucratic* approach – wherein decisions made by professionals are replaced by decisions taken by officials utilising a formal set of rules and regulations. The bureaucratic alternative can be identified with the advantages of a rule-based consistency of decision-making; if the rules and regulations are largely or wholly in the public domain then the bureaucratic approach looks a more effective guarantor of both the 'right to welfare' and the 'right to complain'.

In the context of state welfare, *democratic* procedures may also offer an alternative mode of decision-making about the meeting of needs. Public representatives might in these circumstances take decisions, for example, about the allocation of accommodation or school places, that could otherwise be seen as the purview of housing and education professionals. The democratic alternative can be identified with the traditional advantages claimed for representative democracy – that decisions will reflect 'the views of the community' and that the decision-makers are ultimately accountable to that 'community' through systems of election.

It is of course an over-simplification to refer only to the bureaucratic, and democratic alternatives to professionalism. It is possible to identify other alternatives to individualised professional discretion including market transactions, managerialism, the judicial mode of decision-making, consumerism, voluntarism, and informal caring.

The *market* alternative is often identified with arguments that the professions should be exposed to the rigours of the market-place. There are two points to be made about this. First, what evidence we have of traditional professions (medicine, law) being placed in more market-orientated contexts (for example, doctors and lawyers in the USA) provides little or no evidence that their power or status is much diminished or that professional–client relations are much improved (judging by the volume of medical malpractice suits in the USA). On the other hand, the financial remuneration of the professionals seems to be much enhanced in these circumstances. Secondly, and more significantly, this scenario merely places professions in a different economic context. For market transactions to be a genuine alternative to individualised professional discretion, a decision currently taken by professionals (such as access to prescription drugs) should be replaced by a straightforward consumer transaction (for instance, the same drugs are bought over the counter at a shop with no professional controls exerted over the consumer). The obvious merit of this approach would be to diminish dramatically (and indeed even eliminate) professional controls over non-professionals, allied to the presumed virtues of competitive private markets – competition, choice and efficiency.

The *managerial* alternative involves a transfer of power of key decision-making (especially about resources) to identified individuals who can be made simply and directly accountable through a managerial hierarchy to senior managers and (in state welfare) to public representatives. In the absence of other forms of potentially conflicting authority and controls (peer reviews, codes of ethics, rules and regulations) the manager has the potential, at a stroke, to resolve the problems of accountability associated with 'big government' and 'professionalism' – a way of making democracy work outside the context of parish, rural and urban district councils where the scale of activities precludes the democratic approach identified above.

For a number of key areas (such as child care and mental health) *judicial* modes of decision-making have always been an alternative. Decisions that might be taken by professionals are taken by courts or tribunals. A number of advantages have been claimed for this alternative, most obviously in terms of the clearly defined rights of the individuals about whom decisions are being taken, public knowledge and scrutiny of these decisions, and associated virtues of taking note of the demands of 'natural justice' and 'due process'.

Consumerism implies the empowerment of individual welfare service-users in non-market situations. Decisions that would be taken by professionals are at least subject to greater consumer influence or more radically are transferred to the service-users (or their representatives). This has been advocated in a number of forms including consumer participation or representation within traditional or newly established advisory or decision-making forums (such as school boards of governors, tenant groups) and the creation of quasi-markets (vouchers, parental choice of schools). These may be complemented by a general enhancement of welfare consumer rights. Its advantages seem clear in terms of enhanced individual freedom and control over activities which impinge on people's lives.

Voluntarism implies a reliance on philanthropy and mutual aid to deliver services that might otherwise be identified with the state and with professionals. It should not of course be taken to mean the substitution of 'incompetent amateurs' for 'skilled professionals'. There are well-established traditions of trained volunteers in health and social care (including many forms of counselling and advice work). Advocates of voluntarism as an alternative to professionalism may identify a degree of 'over-training' and 'elitism' with the latter. It may also reflect a degree of faith in personal commitment, and a lack of faith in cash and careerism as a basis for undertaking caring roles. The voluntary alternative combines the virtues of community involvement, freedom from the tyranny of wage-labour and an avoidance of the conspiratorial, power-seeking attributes of professionalism.

Finally the alternative of *informal caring* draws on the roles of families and communities. The greater contemporary significance of this community-based alternative has followed from a growing realisation of the volume of unmet needs with regard to, for example, people with physical disabilities, allied to the awareness of the vast army of informal carers. This alerts us to the presence of a mode of decision-making in which questions about the nature and extent of need are resolved informally by families and neighbours guided by the love and friendship they feel towards the individuals concerned. This approach embodies key qualities (tender loving care) absent from the necessarily socially distant professional approach, It allows for the sort of personalised and if necessary unconventional approach with which professionals cannot, by definition, be associated.

This list of alternatives to professionalism is not intended as exhaustive or definitive. The categories are clearly not self- contained; it would be foolish to pretend that there is, for example, a clear-cut boundary between the informal caring and voluntary roles in welfare. None the less, despite its rather obvious limitations, this categorisation of alternatives to professionalism does indicate a number of crucial points.

First, there are a range of alternatives to traditional forms of professionalism. Secondly, there are a range of advantages associated with these alternatives: for example, the enhancement of individual rights (bureaucratic and judicial alternatives); public scrutiny of key decisions (democratic and judicial alternatives); and consumer and community involvement (consumerism, voluntarism and informal caring). Finally, in any advocacy and defence of interprofessionalism we need to be clear about why we do not simply embrace these alternatives to professionalism and in so doing presumably leave behind for ever all the negative characteristics their critics have identified with the professions.

The alternatives in policy

To what extent has anti-professionalism rhetoric and the availability of alternatives to professionalism been turned into a policy reality? Having attracted an equally vehement volume of critiques it is un-surprising that there are few if any public statements in favour of the bureaucratic approach being preferred to professionalism. It remains to be seen whether the general and growing interest in performance indicators and the specific controls exercised over the education system through the national curriculum and associated testing might be most appropriately categorised as bureaucratic in approach.

Perhaps equally unsurprising, given a tendency for local demo-cratic institutions to fall under the control of opposition parties, there has been little faith in conventional democratic procedures to ameliorate the problems of professionalism. Indeed, in education the potential for charismatic professionals (in the form of dynamic and engaging head teachers) to exercise control has been enhanced in certain respects through the local management of schools and grant-maintained schools.

As already noted, markets have been more obviously used to provide new contexts for, rather than alternatives to, professional-ism. None the less spectacles are more obviously available from garage forecourts and newsagents than was once the case, repre-senting a genuine transfer from the world of professional–client relations to that of retailer–consumer transactions.

The alternative of a managerial approach appears to have been more extensively pursued, especially in the context of health and community care. It could be argued that social care services have become more managerial since the implementation of the recom-mendations of the Seebohm Report (1 April 1971). For the NHS, the significant event was the conclusion of the 'first Griffiths Report' that there was a 'lack of a clearly-defined general management function throughout the NHS' which led to a recommendation that health authorities should identify general managers 'charged with the general management function and overall responsibility for manage-ment's performance in achieving objectives set by the Authority' (DHSS, 1983, p. 11; p. 5). This was accepted by the Government, and from 1 April 1984 the NHS abandoned a system of consensus team management – a form of managerial responsibility which had been based on a perceived need and demand for considerable professional autonomy.

A concern with the implications of extensive professional discretion seemed to be one factor influencing reform of mental health and child care legislation in a manner that has enhanced a judicial approach. The principal changes introduced by the Mental Health Act, 1983 were designed to improve the rights of patients or potential patients; the 1987 White Paper on child care law endorsed the principles that only a court should transfer a parent's legal rights to the local authority, and that a court order is the best method of safeguarding the child's interests (Carrier and Kendall, 1992, pp. 76–8).

The impact of consumerism seems most obvious and most dramatic in education policy, where it is presumed that parental choice of their children's schooling has been significantly enhanced, along with the position and influence of parent governors on school governing bodies.

To what extent successive governments' support for the voluntary sector has enhanced the role of voluntarism is not always easy to discern, given that the most well-known voluntary organisations are themselves the employers of significant numbers of paid and professionally qualified staff.

A growing recognition of informal caring activity has led to attempts to reorder somewhat the perception of the professional role, most obviously through the Barclay Report (1982) where community social work was identified with enabling and supporting informal carers – an attempt to modify and qualify the role of professional social workers as 'front-line providers'. With reference to provision for elderly people the subsequent observation in a government policy paper that care in the community must increasingly mean 'care by the community' (DHSS, 1981, p. 3) seemed indicative of a greater commitment to the informal caring and voluntary sectors.

The alternatives in practice

Whilst it is apparent that the policy agenda has involved an exploration of alternatives to professionalism for a number of years, not all these alternatives have been pursued with equal vigour. In some respects this accords with the content of the critical literature, which tends to be more replete with criticisms of the conventional professionals, than with alternative visions of what might displace these reviled occupations. This may reflect the extent to which some of the alternatives have attracted their own critical literature. There are certainly some well-known and extensive 'problems with' lists that can be attached to the alternatives we explored above.

For example, the bureaucratic alternative looks distinctly unpromising. Bureaucracy has long been associated with 'rigidity' and 'hostility to change'; the phrase 'bureaucratic intraversion' was coined to indicate this hostility, and the tendency for bureaucracies to develop self-justifying routines (Marris and Rein, 1972). This could be linked to Merton's concept of 'ritualism' – 'over-conformity' to rules. The means (bureaucratic rules and regulations) become ends in themselves (Merton, 1968, chs vi and viii). Commentators and consumers have little trouble in identifying this characteristic with social security bureaucracies, especially means-tested public assistance programmes. The resulting web of rigid rules is associated with claimant deterrence, rather than service-user entitlement. So welfare bureaucracies signify routines, rules, regulations, 'red- tape' and rigidity – a set of characteristics that seems certain to militate against innovation, responding to new problems and the sensitive handling of human needs.

Welfare bureaucracy also implies a problem of inequalities in knowledge. The welfare bureaucrats know the rules and regulations which the non-expert consumer struggles to comprehend – a further factor to exclude the latter, even when some needs-based criteria defines them as eligible for services in cash or kind. Issues of inequalities in knowledge figure in another problem of bureaucracy – its anti-democratic bias. It is the officials of the bureaucracy who posses 'expert knowledge'. Can these bureaucracies and their expert, full-time officials be effectively controlled 'in the public interest' by the inexpert public representatives (councillors, MPs, ministers). This problem is particularly serious if the bureaucrats are identified as having a specific set of interests which they pursue independently of 'the public interest'; this indeed is precisely the point developed by the social problem theorists thus:

> the personnel of an organization devoted to a problem tend to build their lives around its continued existence ... they become attached to 'their' problem and anything that threatens to make it disappear or diminish in importance is a threat. (Becker, 1966, Introduction)

Here then is an understandable and identifiable set of interests associated with the welfare bureaucrats: the perpetuation of particular organisations and associated tasks and jobs. A variant of this criticism also surfaced in our separate catalogue of problems associated with professionalism.

Thus both professionalism and bureaucracy may be regarded as posing a rather similar problem for state welfare. They provide us with a situation where there are 'experts' whose knowledge is not widely shared, and where the control of these 'experts' pose considerable difficulties for the 'public representative'. The latter is presumably charged with ensuring state welfare develops in line with 'the public interest'. This conventional assumption of 'democratic control' may obviously be difficult to put into practice in the face of the power and influence of 'the expert'. The 'welfare consumer' may also find it difficult to challenge, complain about and change decisions made by 'experts' either in relation to what is done for a particular individual or decisions which affect a group of people (such as changing the pattern of ante-natal care, closing down a local hospital).

Judicial proceedings have a lengthy if often overlooked welfare history (Carrier and Kendall, 1992, pp. 67–71) but they have not been short of critics and criticisms. In particular conventional court proceedings and 'legalistic approaches' to meeting needs have been questioned in terms of fairness, accessibility, costs, delays, and their adversarial nature (see, for example, Carrier and Kendall, 1992, pp. 71–6). The value of judicial proceedings as an alternative to our characteristically structured welfare services is of course questionable if their effectiveness is in any way dependent on the legal profession and the bureaucracies of the insurance industry.

Informal caring implies a significant role for families and communities, both of which share a conceptual difficulty in that they are no longer taken for granted ways of organising health and social care. While community is the focus of modern care practices, it is nevertheless an idea that has come in for considerable criticism in terms of its components and operational difficulties. Even the family, once an unchallenged institution for the nurture of its members and the meeting of its lifetime needs, is no longer as stable an institution as it was once thought to be.

It is clear that our identifiable alternatives to professionalism come with their own set of potential problems. We may substitute for the discretion of professionals, the discretion of officials, magistrates, judges, councillors, the lay person (jury, voter, volunteer, informal carer) with no hint of a code of ethics to guide the latter. It is often difficult to fathom the basis of professional decision-making and the use of professional discretion. Nevertheless there is a community of professionals, often through regulatory bodies, which have as one of their key objectives the monitoring of discretion in order to avoid abuse, inappropriate dispositions, and unethical behaviour. It is difficult to detect the same set of arrangements that govern the activities of bureaucratic officials, councillors, lay people and even magistrates and judges.

Professional expertise may not be the guarantee of the consistency and uniformity claimed by the professions themselves; but it may generate more consistency of approach than a reliance on lay knowledge, public opinion, the common sense of the judiciary and the principles of politicians.

Ombudsmen-like forms of redress may compensate the individual and judicial review may right an administrative wrong; but the absence of codes of ethics and acceptable professional practice must be a weakness in comparison to those safeguards in professional life. It is noteworthy tht at least for one group of professional public servants, where discretion is often the very essence of their visible role, their published code of professional duties requires them to 'show compassionate respect for the dignity of the individual and to treat every person of whatever social position, race or creed, with courtesy and understanding' (The Metropolitan Police, 1985). We can at least expect some uniformity and consistency of professional knowledge and expertise to be applied to common situations. Variability would have to be justified and defended to peers and tribunals; the bar of public opinion is notoriously arbitrary and not stable enough to provide a bench-mark for meeting needs or redressing complaints.

Professions in the world of welfare

Can state welfare manage without professions? The answer despite the critics and critiques ranged against them, may well be 'no'. Indeed 'to remove the element of professionalism from some services is to remove the rationale for their provision in the first place. That the state is involved in areas of education, health and social care seems to be at least in part to ensure universal access to the professional expertise of teachers, doctors, and nurses; and to prevent the exploitation of the uncertainties and inequalities of knowledge inherent in an activity like health care (Titmuss, 1968, pp. 146–7).

It is also difficult to envisage state welfare operating without some bureaucratic organisation. The concepts of 'rational and efficient decision-making' may geneate the response of 'rational and efficient for whom?' Nevertheless, the rules, regulations and uniformity of treatment associated with bureaucracy can be regarded as essential elements in providing 'rights to welfare'. Is it possible to make adequate provision for citizenship rights without the procedures and practices we associate with bureaucracy?

One conclusion is the necessity to protect professional expertise and skills in order to counter the problems associated with bureaucracy. Another conclusion is that we need those components of bureaucracy – guanteed rights, consistency in the application of rules, justice between those with equal need in the allocation of resources – to provide parameters that can guide and where necessary constrain what could be an excess of professional discretion. So professional activities and bureaucracies present us with a set of potential problems, but do not necessarily prevent the meeting of needs by completely self-interested professional or bureaucratic elites. Furthermore we need a democratic context so that both professionals and bureaucraces are subject to the control and accountability of the polity.

So one answer to one of our opening questions is that state welfare (including health and community care) cannot, without considerable cost, dispense with its long-identified characteristics of bureaucracy and professionalism. In so far as both characteristics have been the subject of much criticism, an appropriate task is to seek out variations on these traditional components of welfare in a manner that minimises their problems and maximises their potential. The issue becomes one not of abandoning professionalism, but rather of getting the best out of it for the consumer and the community (Wilding, 1982, ch. 5).

Conclusions: professional futures and future professionals

Our concern then with the possibilities of interprofessional collaboration has led us through a series of propositions and criticisms of traditional professional practice in order to identify the strengths and weaknesses of the same. The strengths need to be retained and the weaknesses ameliorated. The issue is not the abandonment of professionalism but the means of getting 'the best' out of the tradition for the consumer and the community. This may involve recasting traditional divisions of labour between individualised professional discretion and its alternatives (the decision-making mix), between the more and less professional (the skill mix) and between different professionals (the knowledge mix). The latter two require an interprofessional orientation that looks outside the traditional professional community without abandoning professional ethics and skills.

The decision-making mix

The aim becomes less one of identifying alternatives that may supplant professionalism, but rather one of identifying alternatives that might in some respects complement professionalism. The issue becomes one of the relative roles of professionalism, bureaucracy, democracy and other approaches – an issue we may define as a 'decision-making mix'. The components of this 'mix' may vary between different areas of health and social care. We should not presume that there is an all-encompassing definitive resolution to the problems identified; as others have observed there is no 'single-best solution – if only we were clever enough to find it' (see, for example, Draper *et al.*, 1976).

What might be embraced in such 'decision-making mixes' could be practices designed to make health and social care systems more rather than less open. This could include the promulgation and discussion of rules and regulations by all involved; the building-up of systems of internal review; forms of open administration where freedom of information (without breaching individual client confidentiality) is accepted; the effective representation of the public (properly-paid, full-time representatives with an appropriate degree of back-up facilities); and systems open to some form of audit, inspection, or review. From the judicial approach we might identify the value of independent complaints machinery; and from the consumerist approach we might identify a general commitment to empower service-users.

The skill mix – one meaning of interprofessionalism: the more and less professional

The 'skill mix' issue must involve professionals being willing to accept a form of interprofessionalism which recognises the possibility that some needs may be met as effectively by lesser- trained professionals. Within that possibility lies the potential of a more extensive, accessible service from the same resources with no dilution of quality. Indeed, in so far as it creates the potential for more expensive professional skills to be deployed on tasks for which only they are suitable, a systematic appraisal of skill mixes affords opportunities to enhance service-quality.

The knowledge mix – another meaning of interprofessionalism: the different professions

The 'knowledge mix' involves an understanding that multiprofessional rather than interprofessional relationships have been the norm for many years. Multiprofessionalism involves the retention of specific knowledge but willingness to collaborate across administrative boundaries. What interprofessionalism requires is a willingness to surrender work-roles, to share knowledge and to integrate procedures on behalf of clients.

To succeed in this transition a new form of professional confidence based upon an interprofessional education is urgently required. Such an education will have as its main purpose some of the following features.

1. It will be necessary to share some professional knowledge, for some to be transferred and for some to continue to be claimed and retained as specific to particular groups. The maturity required for such an enterprise can only be built up through a structured interprofessional curriculum. Only from such a base will new knowledge be created and, most importantly, freely communicated.
2. A successful interprofessional education should generate a new form of interprofessional self-awareness, such that those involved will feel to be of equal status with all engaged in the enterprise.
3. Underpinning all such 'new worlds' would be the most important question: for whose benefit is such activity being pursued? While professional self-fulfilment is obviously important, unless the answer without hesitation, is 'the client', then the old criticisms of monopoly and mystification will make their way back on to the scene. We are still dogged by a legacy of health and social care professionals failing to work together. Whether this is to do with the 'deficiencies' of the professional status or the inability of organisations to 'direct' professionals or (the traditional litany of) scarce resources is still an open question.

Two problems are apparent with the agenda associated with interprofessionalism. First, can professionals from different intellectual and vocational backgrounds work together without losing their own specific identities and special skills? Secondly, professional socialisation takes as axiomatic that one of the tasks of professional education is to give future practitioners a strong identity and confidence in competence and practice. Can this be done for interprofessional education?

To instil all this into individuals in a structured manner over a significant period of time produces a reluctance to relinquish that which has been acquired in the course of an uncertain, and in some senses untested, enterprise of collaborative and co-operative working. The entire orientation has been the importance of the individual professional self resorting to colleagues within their own profession for second opinions, psychological support, and confidence in their own competence, rather than to those outside or, worse still, to untutored lay perspectives.

In the end, the three major changes necessary are conceptual, in which knowledge and ethics are rethought; systemic, in which boundaries and practices are stimulated to change, but are not diluted; and methodological, in which the confidence to facilitate, network and evaluate new practice is entered into. Such major changes will necessarily bring with them discussions of the degree of participation of clients in decision-making, the role of the community and the necessity for 'bottom-up' and not just 'top-down' approaches to client needs. This latter may be particularly difficult because of the in-built orientation of most professionals to hold on to their 'strategic' overview (top-down) of the system, in order that the ability to plan the best use of scarce resources is not abandoned in the face of an overload of 'feeling' as the (wrongfully labelled) enemy of rationality. An enormous increase in confidence is required if interprofessional work is to be the norm.

On the surface, such a confidence exists, and the descriptor 'professional' is assumed to give the seal of approval to any occupational activity claiming such a status. Yet such confidence has been attacked for years with critics separated by style, culture, time and continent as diverse as George Bernard Shaw and Ivan Illich. Both have challenged professional dominance. If such an attack can still be mounted, what chance is there for a confident profession to share its intellectual skills, surrender part of its role, allow its boundaries to be crossed by others, potentially lose the claim to best represent the interests of specific clients and co-operate in a loss of status, power and even, eventually, income?

Interprofessional working must not be seen as bowing to the inevitable dilution of skill made necessary by legal and administrative changes, nor must it be based upon an unchallenged acceptance of generalised criticisms of professional practice. If either of these were the reasons for professionals coming together and sharing skills on behalf of clients, the weakness inherent in such motivations would be an unstable and eventually unsustainable base from which to take forward those opportunities offered for making the best of those creditable aspects common to all 'professional' claims. After all, professionals would claim a similar commitment to an ethical code informing all their activities. Such a recognition would render differences in knowledge, practice and work-settings merely fortuitous and not dominant orientations which might adversely affect clients. An interprofessional approach has to be strong enough to allay such fears as may arise from the accuracy of the prediction in the previous sentence, but it also must suggest that interprofessional work is not a form of dilution, rather a stronger set of values and skills which can be harnessed on behalf of clients. Only if such a confidence is engendered will interprofessional collaboration work.

'Hold fast that which is good' (First Epistle of Paul to the Thessalonians, 5:21)

The search for a 'correct view' of professionals is illusory – the 'theoretical history' of the professions is one of varied and conflicting perspectives and evaluations. There is an extensive social science literature on the professions and their place in society. A substantial proportion of this literature is very critical of the professions and professionalisation; they are categorised as devices for acquiring and retaining power, prestige and economic rewards; as subversive to the effective workings of the market to the benefit of consumers; and as a means by which particular social divisions and inequalities are reinforced and sustained. In the social policy literature these issues are associated with a long-standing concern about the power and influence of key professional groups from their input into policymaking at the national level to their relations with service-users and their key roles as arbiters of need and gatekeepers to valued services. Meanwhile, rising expectations related to a number of social and economic changes, including improved living standards and 'more knowledge' – the latter linked to the scope and scale of professional knowledge as well as the influence of the mass media –

seem to have engendered a more critical approach to professionals amongst service-users.

The policy world has often sought to harness professional views to support the policy agenda, but more often than not has found itself in conflict with long-cherished professional values and styles. When policy is translated into bureaucratic health and social care delivery systems, the stage is set for a conflict between values based upon professional discretion and judgement and bureaucratic rules based upon accountability and the responsibility for rationing scarce resources. If professionals define 'need' and bureaucratic officials control resources to meet needs, the claim that interprofessional collaboration will break any deadlock resulting from the definition being held by one group and the distribution being held by another requires careful scrutiny.

Community care policies require interprofessional contacts of some sort and the advent of the health and community care refos in the 1990s brings to the fore long-standing issues germane to the quality of care the users of health and social care services can expect to receive. There is the place of the professional within public service bureaucracies – which includes the new health and social care providers created by the purchaser–provider splits in health and community care. There is also the relationship between different professionals and those with different skills, located in different agencies.

What happens to professional loyalty when solo practice is no longer the norm and the client is no longer the object of total professional concern? Can professionals be loyal to employing health and social care providers where concerns with administrative and economic efficiency may appear to take precedence over the priorities as defined by the profession and the professionals?

There are also the uncertain relationships consequent upon the changing boundaries of work and role which have followed the administrative and legal changes of the 1980s and 1990s in health and community care. This is particularly important with reference to the relationship between doctors, nurses and social workers and between these professions, 'semi-professions' and other health and social care personnel over shared clients. Such relationships will almost certainly involve implicit, if not explicit, judgements about old and new territories, competencies, legal authority, accountability and personal autonomy.

An interprofessional agenda for the year 2000 should at least be conscious of the previous criticisms of professional identity and practice. At the same time such consciousness should embrace an interprofessional approach to client needs, which holds fast to those features of professional life which have defended client needs and given well-deserved honour (and we use this term rather than that of 'status' deliberately) to those whose life's work has been to uphold the best in professional practice.

We therefore take issue with the spirit, but not the purpose or form expressed by Vita Sackville-West in her praise of the yeoman farmer:

> Few words must serve his turn.
> For he's sagacious who lives taciturn.
> And airs no noisy cunning of his trade,
> But keeps his private purpose deeply laid;
> Gives neighbours nothing of his confidence,
> And takes his counsel of his own good sense.
> No wise man utters what he inly knows;
> Certainty in a loose uncertain world
> Is far too firm a treasure, wiseman goes
> Jealous and wary, keeping darkly furled
> His small particular knowledge . . .

> (Vita Sackville West, 'Winter', from *The Land*,
> Heinemann, London, 1926, p. 22)

References

Abel-Smith, B. (1964), *The Hospitals, 1800–1948: a study in social administration in England and Wales* (London: Heinemann).

Audit Commission (1986), *Making a Reality of Community Care: a report* (HMSO: London).

Barclay Report (Chair: Peter Barclay) (1982), *Social workers: their role and tasks* (London: Bedford Square Press).

Becker, H. (1966), *Social Problems: a modern approach* (Wiley: Chichester).

Butler-Sloss Report (Chair: Lord Justice Butler-Sloss) (1988), *Report of the Inquiry into Child Abuse in Cleveland* (London: HMSO).

Carrier, J. and Kendall, I. (1992) 'Law and the social division of welfare', *International Journal of the Sociology of Law*, vol. 20, pp. 61–87 (London: Academic Press).

Day, P. and Klein, R. (1987), *Accountabilities: five public services* (London: Tavistock).

DHSS (1970), *National Health Service: the Future Structure of the National Health Service* (London: HMSO).

DHSS (1981), *Growing Older*, Cmnd. 8173 (London: HMSO).

DHSS (1983), *NHS Management Inquiry Report* (Griffiths Report) (London: DHSS).

Department of Health (1989a), *Working for Patients*, CM555 (London: HMSO).

Department of Health (1989b), *Caring for People: community care in the next decade and beyond*, CM 849 (London: HMSO).

Draper, P., Grenholm, G. and Best, G. (1976), 'The organization of health care: a critical view of the 1974 reorganization', in D. Tuckett (ed.), *An Introduction to Medical Sociology* (London: Tavistock).

Etzioni, A. (ed.) (1969), *The semi-professions and their organization: teachers, nurses, social workers* (New York: Free Press).

Freidson, E. (1986), *Professional powers: a study of the institutionalisation of formal knowledge* (Chicago: University of Chicago Press).

Griffiths, R. (1988), *Community care: agenda for action: a report to the Secretary of State for Social Services* (London: HMSO).

Hughes, M. Mayall, B., Moss, P., Perry, J., Petrie, P., and Pinkerton, G. (1980), *Nurseries Now: a fair deal for parents and children* (Harmondsworth: Penguin).

Illich, I. (1978), *The right to useful unemployment and its professional enemies* (London: Boyars).

Jones, K. (1972), *A History of the Mental Health Services* (London: Routledge & Kegan Paul).

Jones, K. (1983), in P. Bean and S. MacPherson (eds), *Approaches to Welfare* (London: Routledge & Kegan Paul).

Colwell Report (1974), *Report of the Committee of Inquiry into the Care and Supervision Provided in Relation to Maria Colwell* (Chair: T. G. Field-Fisher) (London: HMSO).

Marris, P. and Rein, M. (1972), *Dilemmas of Social Reform: poverty and community action in the United States* (London: Routledge & Kegan Paul).

Marshall, T. H. (1963), *Sociology at the crossroads and other essays* (London: Heinemann).

Merton, R. (1968), *Social Theory and Social Structure* (enlarged edition), (New York: Free Press).

The Metropolitan Police (1985), *The Principles of Policing and Guidance for Professional Behaviour* (London: Metropolitan Police).

Ministry of Health (1968), *National Health Service: The Administrative Structure of the Medical and Related Services in England and Wales* (London: HMSO).

National Development Group for the Mentally Handicapped (1976), *Mental Handicap: Planning Together* (London: DHSS/HMSO).

Nokes, P. (1967), *The Professional Task in Welfare Practice* (London: Routledge & Kegan Paul).

Redcliffe-Maud Report (1969), Royal Commission on Local Government in England, Report, Volume One, Cmnd. 4040 (Chair: Sir John Redcliffe-Maud) (London: HMSO).

Royal Commission on the NHS (1978), Research Paper No. 1: *The working of the National Health Service* (London: HMSO).

Royal Commission on the NHS (1979), (Chairman: Sir Alec Merrison) Cmnd. 7615, (London: HMSO).

Seebohm Report (1968), *Report of the Committee on Local Authority and Allied Personal Social Services* (Chair: Sir Frederic Seebohm), Cmnd. 3703 (London: HMSO).

Social Services Committee (1985), Second report, Session 1984–85, Community Care with special reference to adult mentally ill and mentally handicapped people, 13–1 (London: HMSO).

Titmuss, R. M. (1968), *Commitment to Welfare* (London: George Allen & Unwin).

Ward, C., (1976) *Housing: an anarchist approach* (London: Freedom Press).

Wilding, P. (1982), *Professional power and social welfare* (London: Routledge & Kegan Paul).

Wilensky, H. and Lebeaux, C. (1965), *Industrial Society and Social Welfare: the impact of industrialisation on the supply and organization of social welfare services in the United States* (New York: The Free Press).

Willcocks, A. (1967), *The creation of the National Health Service: a study of pressure groups and a major social policy decision* (London: Routledge & Kegan Paul).

2 *Professionals and management*

Patricia Owens and Heather Petch

Chapter summary

This chapter continues and elaborates the themes addressed in Chapter 1. The changes in the NHS and social services are examined with reference to the profound effects on the structure and function of professional groups such as nurses, doctors and social workers. Drawing upon their own original research over the last decade, the authors discuss the impact of the introduction of general management, the allocation of budgets to services, the development of internal market principles and the purchaser–provider division. The accumulative effect has been to dismantle traditional professional hierarchies and radically to change accepted patterns of care.

Whom do they serve?

Most professionals in health and social services work in large formal organisations. This means that they are employed either in a clinical or an expert role to perform certain tasks, and/or they are involved in service management, as has been discuss in Chapter 1 by Carrier and Kendall. The professions have always posed problems of definition for classical writers on organisational theory, as their autonomous status and presence within bureaucratic and formalised structures creates the potential for conflict. Analysts of the management of organisations have tended to ignore the professionals within, and sociologists have similarly paid little attention to the organisations in which they work, or have portrayed them as antithetical to professional values. The separate and different educational backgrounds and socialisation of managers and professional groups has reinforced these problems of co-existence.

Max Weber (1947) described the classic system of bureaucratic control as having four fundamental characteristics: these are hierarchy, continuity, impersonality, and rule by experts. This ideal type of organisation had clearly defined divisions of labour, each level being accountable to the one above. This pattern created a career structure, and job security. To ensure impartiality the system functioned according to prescribed rules, and experts were trained to perform specific tasks in accordance with these prescriptions (Bendix, 1977). Weber's model was structured to maximise rationality and technical efficiency. But critics have said that there are problems with such organisations, as rules can become inflexible, impersonality can become indifference, and too much hierarchy can discourage individuals from developing a sense of personal responsibility and initiative. Beatham (1987) suggested that Weber failed to realise the ambivalent nature of bureaucratic structures. Individual professionals have to act at a personal level with a client or patient, and at the same time relate to the formal structure of the organisation in which they are employed. Inevitably this causes some tensions as the rules governing individual and corporate behaviour may be at odds with each other.

The 'iron cage' of bureaucracy that Weber described has been modified by subsequent writers, who have identified the informal networks that exist between professionals, and the strong element of individual discretion that comes into play (Blau, 1972). During training professionals develop their own set of norms and values: examples of this process are described in *Learning and Working: The Occupational Socialization of Nurses* (Melia, 1987), and *The Boys in White: Student Culture in Medical School* (Becker *et al.*, 1960).

Students in these professions traditionally have been educated in isolation in medical or nursing schools separated from the general undergraduate population, and this has had an important impact on the development of tribal attitudes after qualification. *Project 2000: A New Preparation for Practice* (UKCC, 1986) is an important step in nurse education which aims to address this problem and integrate nurses more fully into the mainstream of tertiary education. However, once they are employed in a public service system, they also have to incorporate the broader aims and objectives of larger organisations, and this may mean that conflicts develop between corporate and individual professional goals.

Bureaucracies also develop their own cultures with elaborate codes governing the behaviour of employees, and there are shared assumptions about the aims of the organisation (Peters and Waterman, 1982). Public bureaucracies sometimes perceive themselves as guardians of the national interest: there is the idea that they embody ideals that transcend policies of particular governments, they can develop a character of their own, become set in their ways and difficult to change. The 'iron cage' of bureaucracy could in fact act to protect the public interest or alternatively to prevent innovation and change.

Most public service systems such as the NHS are monopolistic, and hitherto there has been little pressure from the market to change the ways of professionals within them to increase efficiency. Also, consumers have difficulty in taking their business elsewhere. In the absence of external sanctions, such bureaucratic organisations run the risk of becoming self-serving, because power is vested in individual control of scarce resources, and the focus is not necessarily on outcomes (Drucker, 1979). In these circumstances, professionals can be more concerned with their own survival than with the broader aims of providing for the needs of consumers of their services.

A world apart

Carrier and Kendall in Chapter 1 have outlined the growing power and influence of the numerous occupational groups within our social and health care systems. The professional is characterised by the acquisition of skills based on theoretical knowledge, specialist training, tests of competence, belonging to an independent organisation, possessing specific codes of conduct and ethics of altruistic service. The model of the medical professional has strongly influenced the structures developed by other professional or aspiring semi-professional groups which also have adopted statutory governing bodies for licensing, standard-setting and autonomous status.

The idea of professions as self-regulating groups that are altruistic has been challenged by writers such as Friedman (1962) and Mueller (1979), who dismiss it as fiction, and say that it is more accurate to describe their activities as expressions of restrictive practices. Monopolising knowledge, restricting entry, and setting a high price for services, can be viewed as protection or exploitation of the consumers. The cloak of specialist knowledge can be interpreted merely as a disguise to win resource battles, or to exercise group power politics. A less jaundiced view is that standard-setting gives the public a sense of security in their dealings with professionals. However, it is clear there are two sides to the professional coin.

Etzioni (1969) suggested that there was a conflict between the structural and sanctioned values of organisations and the core values that professionals internalise during training. But claims to professional high status and disinterested dedication are, to some extent, measures that uphold and legitimise the protection from the labour market that they seek (Atkinson, 1983).

There are many different professional or semi-professional groups in health and social care, and hitherto they have each been ordered vertically and hierarchically, and have had a tendency to have a primary loyalty to their own group, and not to the organisation itself (Davies, 1983). The need for central administrative systems in large bureaucratic enterprises is at odds with the professionals stress on decentralisation and personal decision-making. Scott and Myer (1983) suggested that the conflict lies between the managers emphasising macro-criteria and professionals and practitioners focusing on micro-criteria.

Take me to your leader

In October 1983, Roy Griffiths, Deputy Chairman and Managing Director of Sainsbury's, wrote a letter to the Secretary of State for Health and Social Services, the Rt Hon. Norman Fowler MP. In it he outlined proposals for the complete and radical restructuring of the NHS. The central idea was to introduce general managers at every level to run the services. They would replace the interprofessional consensus management teams that had been collectively responsible for taking decisions since 1974. Each part of the NHS would be led by an individual manager.

The decision to adopt the recommendations in the letter was far from popular with professional groups. The nurses saw such changes as an assault on their hard-won victories a decade earlier, when they had gained representation at every level of decision-making in the NHS (Owens and Glennerster, 1990). There were several major themes in the Griffiths letter. These were first, that the service needed leadership and to agree priorities; secondly, that more attention should be given to value for money; thirdly, that professionals should be accountable to managers; and fourthly, that management should be devolved to smaller units of service delivery.

The late Tom Evans, Director of the King's Fund College summarised the thrust of the changes as a transformation of the organisation of the NHS from one that was administrative and professional in character to one with a managerial culture. The most often quoted passage in the Griffiths letter was, 'In short, if Florence Nightingale were carrying her lamp through the corridors of the NHS today, she would almost certainly be looking for the people in charge' (para 5).

I win, you lose

The NHS had developed a structure based on separately managed and distinct occupational groups. It was conceived as a coalition between these professional entities. The Salmon Report (1966) described managing the care of the patient as 'many people working together', with 'managers of each major function', and 'their duty is to control their subordinates'. It was not thought necessary to put any one person in charge of a service as a whole, and this was underpinned by the belief that any conflict could be resolved by discussion and negotiation between professionals.

These concepts rested on ideas of personal collaboration, not on authority structures and formal bureaucratic hierarchies (Beatham, 1987). They were embodied in the 'Grey Book' (DHSS, 1972) which objected to putting one person in charge, and advocated multidisciplinary teams, through which managers and professionals 'can jointly make decisions' (para 1:24). Decisions needed the agreement of all team members, but in the harsh economic climate of the 1980s this system began to run into trouble, as it was ill-adapted to make difficult choices. Griffiths argued that the inability to resolve conflicts by reaching agreement by consensus was leading to organisational inertia (Owens and Glennerster, 1990).

Informal patterns of collaboration had been crucial to the way the health service worked, but the Grey Book played down the importance of conflict and the seriously negative and damaging outcomes of failure to agree decisions. In conditions of more and more pressure on limited resources, the 'zero sum games' played by professionals meant increasingly occurring situations of 'impasse', where advances by one could only be made at the expense of another.

Competition between professional groups had been firmly related to the budgets over which they held sway. Success was not measured in terms of the quality of the service provided, but more crudely in terms of the size of the budget they could command (Drucker, 1979). Separate professional hierarchies naturally like to see the world from their own profession's point of view, and this made a corporate strategy difficult to achieve in the old consensus model of NHS management. The introduction of general management and subsequent reorganisation of the NHS into a corporate structure stimulated open power struggles between dominant professional groups such as administrators, doctors and nurses (Owens and Glennerster, 1990). The fierce struggles played out by the nursing profession at this time give an insight into the importance of these issues for all professional groups who worked within the system, and who valued their autonomous status.

The 'Garden of Eden' complex

In January 1986 the Royal College of Nursing mounted a national advertising campaign in the press, opposing the introduction of general management. The advertisements showed Florence Nightingale along-side a modern nurse, with a caption that suggested that the ancestor of nursing's standards of care were to be compromised. Another showed a manager with a calculator, and suggested that he did not 'know his coccyx from his humerus', and by inference was only interested in cost and not patients. These advertisements were stark illustrations of the gulf of understanding between one professional group and another in the NHS. They also indicated professionals at that time did not think it was necessarily their business to know about or consider cost, or managers to have an understanding of the service in which they worked. The advertisement included a form which asked readers to sign a statement which read, 'I agree that nursing should be run by nurses'.

This was an illustration of the tribal and self-governing nature of nursing in particular, but also of professional groups in general. They did not represent themselves predominantly as part of the NHS system composed of a multiplicity of different professionals who work together to produce a total service for patients. The hidden agenda was the fear that the Griffiths' proposals would dismantle the Salmon (1966) nurse management structure, fought for long and hard, which had achieved parity for nurses with administrators and the medical professional, with nurse managers at every level (Owens and Glennerster, 1990).

The need for equal status in the administrative structure had a long and complex history, as up to a point it was closely connected to gender differences, sexual politics and division of labour between professional groups in the NHS. Some writers have suggested that the pattern which developed was derived from the health care systems of the past. Professional relationships inside hospitals reflected the Victorian patriarchal family ideal, where female nurses were perceived as mothers and carers, and male doctors as fathers, with patients as dependent children (Game and Pringle, 1983; Garmanikow, 1978).

Salvage (1985) described how these stereotyped ideas characterised the power relations in hospitals and bureaucratic domination. A study of the NHS workforce revealed that although 75 per cent was female, 91 per cent of managers were men (Chiplin and Sloane, 1982). In nursing 43–50 per cent of management posts were occupied by men, although they only constituted 10 per cent of the workforce, and only 3 per cent in inner London (Davies and Rosser, 1986). The move towards general management was therefore viewed with some anxiety by nurses, as it seemed a step in the wrong direction from the point of view of women's access to positions of power within the new general management order.

In addition, a growing militancy also emerged that exposed the open divide between the RCN and the other unions, COHSE and NUPE. Jane Salvage wrote in *The Politics of Nursing* (1985), that a new radicalism was, in part, a response to the tougher management styles emerging in the health service due to the increasing pressures on budgets and the search for cheaper ways to deliver care. This latter development threatened the status and integrity of nurses and other professional groups by opening the way to new ideas about the delivery of care and blurring the boundaries between professional groups.

In these circumstances, nurses had the advantage of being able to call upon their ancestor Florence Nightingale to promote their cause in the twentieth century. Groups hold together over time using the powerful vehicles of myth and ritual (Lévi-Strauss, 1977: Malinowski, 1974). Conceptions of the past and the activities of the present are usually associated with some explanation about the genesis of the group and its genitor. Usually, ancestors epitomise the principal group ideology and serve to symbolise the structure of that collectivity. By tracing lineage from a particular ancestor, descendants can validate claims about 'property' or 'knowledge' or a specific 'moral' code in terms of a definable past focused on a particular person or natural symbol. Organisations or groups work like this to hold together over time in an abstract as well as a physical sense (Douglas, 1987).

However, one of the problems with the ancestry of nursing is that the whole profession does not owe its origins to Florence Nightingale. In the past, nurses in the poor law hospitals were often recruited from the pauper inhabitants, and similarly those who worked in the asylums were poor and uneducated. These two groups of nurses ultimately formed the basis of COHSE, and were prepared to strike. Many followers of the other nursing organisations such as the RCN initially believed that these attitudes undermined their quest for respectability and status as a profession, and divided nursing.

Nurses' internal struggles and external battles for equal status with doctors and administrators, like other professionals working in the highly formalised structure of the NHS, became diverted and preoccupied with issues such as power over their own budgets and workforce. But the use of the Nightingale myth in the campaign against general management was supremely inappropriate, and showed a misunderstanding of her life and work. In fact, historians have described her in terms that could be adopted for many a modern chief executive, certainly not in those applicable to the post-Salmon nurse manager. The exclusivity of the professional in functional management is actually a twentieth- century phenomenon.

Strachey (1918) wrote that 'the gentle vision of female virtue' was in reality a potent driving force, reorganising kitchens and laundries in army hospitals, and supervising the building of wards, ventilation, drains and sewers, supplies of medicine, beds and clothing. In her own words nursing was, 'the least important of the functions into which she had been forced'. Strachey described her filling papers with recommendations and suggestions, criticising in detail the organisation, calculating contingencies, with exhaustive analyses and statistical statements 'piled up in breathless eagerness one on top of the other'. She attacked incompetent doctors, self-sufficient nurses and inert officials with 'the deadly precision of a machine gun', and was altogether a different being from the traditional stereotype of ministering angel.

It could be argued that the holistic model of nursing care that Florence Nightingale developed in the nineteenth century, far from being sullied by the introduction of general management, actually helped to revive some of its core values which had been distorted and overlaid by subsequent generations of nurses. By introducing budgets for services, with responsibility placed in one manager, the vertical and hierarchical management and financial control structures based on professional groups which characterised the NHS, were swept away.

Ultimately, many nurses welcomed the changes, and gladly let go of their exclusively professional roles to take on general management (Owens and Glennerster, 1990). They brought to general management the additional benefit of their clinical expertise. However, in 1993 there is still concern about the lack of women in general management posts, and NHS management are making strenuous efforts to remedy this situation by providing equal opportunities for the future (NAHAT, 1993–4).

Will you, won't you, join the dance?

In the years that have followed the implementation of the Griffiths' proposals the movement of professionals into management has been dramatic, and nurses have been foremost in taking on general management roles at all levels of the health service. Griffiths also recommended the allocation of budgets for doctors leading clinical teams in hospitals: it was proposed that clinicians be given responsibility for resources that would cover all activity within a unit of hospital service as clinical directors. This was clearly a measure that would involve doctors in the future in the financial aspects of care and control of expenditure.

Initially there was huge resistance to this initiative, and few clinicians opted to become general managers, but clinical directorates headed up by doctors are now becoming the norm rather than the exception in the 1990s. In addition, the introduction of clinical audit to study effectiveness of treatments and outcome within professional groups and in multidisciplinary teams was to become an important tool for the management process, to improve efficiency, performance and quality.

But the problem was that up until the late 1980s no one in the health service had a clear idea of how much services cost. The Resource Allocation Working Party (RAWP), using a formula based on population statistics, had operated to provide funds at Regional and District levels. In April 1989 the Conservative government embarked on a programme of far-reaching and radical reforms in health and social care. 'Working for Patients' was a blueprint for developing a new system for allocating and controlling budgets, and there was a dramatic shift towards a contract culture. A boundary was introduced between those who purchased and those who provided health care. The objectives set out in these working papers were later incorporated into the NHS and Community Care Act 1990.

The reforms had profound implications for primary health care. It had been recognised by the politicians that GPs were the gatekeepers to secondary and tertiary care, and for this reason the Family Practitioner Committees (FPCs) who had been left out of the first round of

Griffiths' proposals in 1984 were drawn into the general management philosophy as well. Their name was changed to Family Health Services Authorities (FHSAs), and the administrative culture was also transformed into a management- style organisation in line with other parts of the NHS.

The most important change was the introduction of the purchaser and provider split. This meant that in the future, the direct management role of the District Health Authorities was changed into a commissioning agency structure to purchase services. There was no longer a direct management role at district level, and all hospitals and community services in the NHS were encouraged and finally instructed to form Trusts and become self-governing bodies providing health care. Within the commissioning authorities, health care professionals play a central role in identifying health needs of local populations and deciding how to spend budgets in the most appropriate and equitable way. Many professionals have direct management responsibility as chief executives, executive directors of boards of commissioning authorities or Trusts, or as managers of units of service. A high proportion of these roles are combinations of the clinical and management dimensions of care. Professionals have gradually become integrated into the corporate structure, and work in multidisciplinary teams at all levels, usually led by a general manager who combines responsibility for both clinical standards and financial control.

Although the FHSAs had been drawn into the management structures, and joint purchasing arrangements include DHAs and Social Services, GPs still remained outside, as they have independent contractual status. The new reforms were aimed at drawing GPs into the new corporate ethos of the NHS. The problem was that although constraints could be imposed on GPs, they were not directly employed by the health service, and it was therefore much more difficult to introduce the idea of general management. The size and scale of the NHS was evident in large institutions like District General Hospitals, but was not so obvious to GPs working in very small units of service. (A more detailed analysis of the evolution of the modern primary health care team is to be found in Chapter 9.) But it was this small business approach to health care and the individualistic and entrepreneurial ethos of many GPs that the reformers saw as a possible avenue for influencing and ultimately radically changing their culture.

Titmuss (1968) identified the crucial role of GPs in the NHS as the co-ordinators of care and the initiators of every train of causation which led to the use of sophisticated hospital medical care. The government, in their drive to control rising costs in health care, recognised the major role that GPs had as rationers of care, weighing individual patient needs, and determining their priority of access to the full spectrum of specialist care (Butler and Calnan, 1988). With these things in mind, they incorporated some important innovations into the new package of reforms in the *Working for Patients* papers.

One of the most revolutionary of these innovations was the introduction of budgets for general practice. GPs with over 9000 patients were invited to become fundholders for their patients for treatments that were non-emergency and for a prescribed list of standard procedures. Later the budget covered care in the community as well. This was a completely new idea, derived in part from the models in the USA of Health Maintenance Organisations (HMOs) which were managed by doctors. However, there were considerable differences, as the HMOs were funded on an individual patient basis through occupational pensions or some means-tested state benefits such as Medicaid or Medicare, whereas the UK scheme had no formula to assist in assessing budgets on a capitation or per-patient basis for individual general practice populations. In the absence of earmarked funds *per capita* for each patient, Regions simply assessed budgets by relying on past patterns of referral to hospital services, although before long an average annual cost per-patient began to emerge across the Regions. Also introduced at this time was the concept of 'indicative prescribing', a system in which FHSAs allocated a budget for drugs to all practices after discussion with the GPs, and encouraged generic prescribing and monitoring of expenditure.

The outcome of these two major changes has meant that to a greater or lesser degree all GPs have suddenly found themselves at the sharp end of resource management. After the introduction of fundholding in some areas 50 per cent of a District budget for non-emergency work was being managed by GPs. Glennerster *et al.* in the King's Fund Institute study (1992), found that the first wave of GPs who volunteered for fundholding in 1990 were those who had a high degree of management expertise and organisational flair already. Doctors who were enthusiastic demonstrated that they could take the challenge of resource management in their stride.

Critics of the scheme complained that non-fundholding practice patients were suffering a disadvantage, as fundholders were able to buy services in a more flexible way across District boundaries, and gain favourable access to waiting lists. This posed ethical problems in terms of determining the equitable distribution of resources across the population, and these important dilemmas remain to be re-solved. However, the scheme demonstrated the capacity of GPs to manage resources and find more effective and efficient ways of meeting their patients' needs. A more general discussion of these issues is set out in Chapter 3.

A further outcome was the changes that occurred to interprofes-sional relationships. The practice manager became a key figure in the new reforms, not only to process all the monitoring exercises and target setting for GPs and FHSAs, but also to play a central and proactive role in the management of resources and patient referrals. These posts are now attracting a new kind of person, many come from commercial backgrounds and bring a different perspective to the organisation of primary health care teams.

Another important outcome was the profound change in relation-ships between consultants and GPs. After 1947 and the creation of the NHS, this intraprofessional divide had become more profound, with the GPs taking on the role of the 'poor relation' although this situation has gradually improved since 1964 (see Chapter 9 for a full history). In the past, GPs had felt powerless to influence what hap-pened to patients once they were referred to hospital, but now their status as purchasers gave them the capacity to 'exit' a service if it did not meet the requirements of their patients. This had the effect of encouraging GPs and consultants to meet and discuss their services in a much more focused way than in the past, although the resent-ments of consultants were and are played out in constant debates in the press and media.

Some fundholders invited consultants to see patients at their prac-tice premises, thus developing a closer relationship. Like the nur-ses, many of the arguments about management changes were intimately concerned with the relative power and status *within* pro-fessional groups, and *internal* professional rivalries about control of resources. Both intraprofessional and interprofessional relationships in the medical profession were fundamentally altered by the intro-duction of fundholding to a degree that had not been anticipated at the outset, as GPs became the prioritisers and rationers for their group of patients.

Where are they now?

Nursing and social work in the community also did not escape the shock-waves of reform. The Cumberlege Report (1983) argued that community nursing was in a rut, 'shackled by out-moded role de-marcations and rigid work patterns'. There was poor liaison inter-nally between community nurses, and externally with other primary health care professionals, social services and hospitals. Underpinning these criticisms was a management vacuum which was to be filled by the proposed patch-based system for community nursing.

Locality nursing became the model widely adopted in the 1980s. However, the reforms outline in *Working for Patients* and *Caring for People* has stimulated changes to the occupational boundaries be-tween health and social care. Community nurses may have some of their traditional role taken over by higher profile practice nurses, home care assistants, specialist outreach nurses or link-workers, and the new care and assessment managers based in social services departments.

The cost-containment culture has put all professional roles under new scrutiny. The establishment of different self-govern-ing Trusts free from the constraints imposed by the Whitley scales of payment for health care staff, may further lead to a fragmenta-tion of the workforce. GP fundholders may prefer to use practice nursing staff for their own community-based work in the future, thus breaking down entirely the concept of management hierar-chies based on occupational groupings in the community. Many tasks hitherto defined as nursing may be delegated to less skilled-workers.

There is some anxiety that radical changes in the skill-mix of primary health care teams could only serve to weaken the service by diluting specialist functions. The heavy emphasis on child health surveillance and immunisations in health promotion targets has, in theory, increased the responsibility of the health visitors. However, GPs may prefer in the future to cover this aspect of health care using their own practice-based nurses rather than practice-attached staff employed and managed by Trusts (Petch and Owens, 1993). If this happens, it will inevitably affect and change the roles and inter-pro-fessional relationship between community health and social care staff.

But moving away from a specialist to a more generic approach in nursing in the community is in counterpoint to what is happening in social services. Both *Caring for People* and 'The Children Act 1989' reinforce a move towards specialisation within local authority social care services. The introduction of compulsory competitive tendering and the purchaser–provider split have also influenced skill-mix changes. Child care and protection responsibilities could be contracted out to private or voluntary organisations, even though the statutory responsibility remains with the local authority. Some local authorities are moving less towards the generic case worker model, and more towards a system of defined care groups and specialist care managers who will assess their clients' general needs.

By introducing these changes, the government has replaced the monopoly of the statutory services and introduced a more dominant role for the voluntary sector as service providers. This is intended to encourage greater range and flexibility in social care. The statutory services are recast as 'enablers' and, paralleling developments in the NHS, they have become commissioners and definers of appropriate services to meet the identified needs of people in the community. They will be providing direct services less and less, and social services professionals will find themselves more and more working in organisations outside the public sector.

However, the underlying belief that the voluntary and private sector will necessarily provide a more flexible and innovative service may be misplaced. Voluntary organisations which are small, and often staffed by unpaid workers, in practice have to become more like the statutory services if they are to deal with the expansion created by new demands. Ironically, the voluntary organisations could become as rigid and bureaucratic as the statutory services they are intended to replace (Kramer, 1981).

In theory, at least, the creation of joint commissioning and multidisciplinary working recognises the importance of professionals cooperating across boundaries. But with different and separate management structures still in existence, it is difficult to see how the neater and tidier Griffiths' concept of general management and clinical directorates characteristic of the hospital sector can work as efficiently out in the community services where competition is rife, and a thousand flowers boom.

Professionals in the future will find themselves working in a wide variety of organisations outside the public sector. Community nurses are currently employed by Trusts, but could in the future be employed directly by fundholding GPs; local authority community care staff are often performing similar functions to NHS nurses; and some specialists, such as health visitors, are threatened by practice nurses extending their roles in the field of child health surveillance. In the fields of mental health, learning disabilities and homelessness, care and assessment managers and staff are recruited from a wider variety of social and health care professional backgrounds and are not exclusively social workers.

'Things fall apart; the centre cannot hold'

'The falcon cannot hear the falconer' ('The Second Coming', Yeats, 1921). This chapter has described the effect of a decade of reform and organisational change that has been unprecedented since the foundation of the NHS in 1948. Professional hierarchies and power bases have been challenged in the process. The Conservatives favoured the Friedmanite economic principles as set out in *Capitalism and Freedom* (1982). These were firmly grounded in a competitive market philosophy governed by contractual relationships. They were designed to promote private enterprise, limit the scope of government and control public expenditure, and are reflected in recent changes to our welfare services. The accumulative effect has been to dismantle professional hierarchies and disperse their power bases. This process has been observed on both sides of the Atlantic, and mirrors the fate of the unions in many of the nationalised industries after privatisation.

The question is whether this is a strategy that increases the freedom of the patient or client to have equal access to high quality welfare services. In other words, if the demands of consumers determine the shape of the market, does it provide a more flexible and equitable service than one subject to a rational planning and with distribution processes based on the knowledge and skills of professional groups?

Friedman suggested that the overthrow of the medieval guild system was an early step in the rise of freedom in the Western world, and a triumph of liberal ideas. He perceived the increasing tendency to licence to practice particular occupations as a retrograde step, and contended that professional monopolies limited the possibilities of experimentation. His argument for the market, even in the field of health care was that it had 'a tolerance of diversity', and 'an ability to utilize a wide range of special knowledge and capacity'. He concluded that: 'It renders special interest groups impotent to prevent experimentation and permits the customer and not the producers to decide what will serve the customers best.' But, as the market is an impersonal force, there will be winners and losers, and the weaker members of society may not gain a fair share, but Friedman argued that rational planning by professionals did not guarantee fair shares anyway.

This chapter has described the consequences for professional hierarchies of the introduction of general management, service budgets, the split between purchasers and providers in health and welfare services, and the devolution of service provision for many priority groups to the private and voluntary sector. This has ultimately resulted in the dismantling of professional frameworks, a strong movement towards privatising the labour force, and increased fragmentation of welfare services. Constant change and reorganisation has also limited the professionals' capacity to develop rational planning systems over the long term.

By reducing professional roles in this way to those of purveyors of goods, there is a serious risk of eroding their value and status in society, and, along with it, professionals' commitment and sense of altruism. These ethics of service are difficult to quantify but need to be accepted. If we dismiss them entirely, as Friedman does, we may end up knowing the price of everything and the value of nothing, and our health and welfare services will be diminished – if not our whole society.

In the early part of this chapter, we described Douglas's ideas about the capacity of modern organisations to fix their belief systems upon natural symbols such as ancestors, illustrating their use by ascriptive groups like nurses and doctors to bring the past into the present. Her scholarly analysis *How Institutions Think* tells us that organisations are not thinking independently or necessarily with common purpose, and cannot build themselves. They are, she suggests, the sum of the people within them and their thoughts and values. This is particularly the case for welfare institutions, as underlying them are the humanitarian beliefs of the ancestors of medicine and nursing (in particular, Hippocrates and Florence Nightingale) and more recently the collectivist beliefs of William Beveridge and Bevan are at their core. Often incoherently expressed, by politicians of all persuasions, but firmly adhered to, is the principle of a comprehensive and free NHS (Klein, 1983).

The new market-oriented NHS and social service departments, liberated – in Friedman's terms – from the spirit of collectivism, may have cast professionals adrift into a universe of uncertainty. Douglas suggests that institutions can remember but also systematically forget: 'competitive social systems are weaker on memory than ascriptive ones', she wrote, 'driving out some players and bringing others to the top'. With each organisational change public memory becomes weakened and the past rearranged to fit in with the present. Professional traditions can become obscured by the dilution of their power bases and, in the process, the principles of service which underpinned their commitment to professional standards can be undermined, if all caring is reduced to a simple financial transaction.

But there remains a pressure towards developing coherent principles of organisation. Douglas contends that to accomplish change it is necessary to amalgamate and rationalise the justificatory stories of the past as part of this process. The proposed corporate governance strategy for the NHS appears to be a step in this direction. Its purpose is to 'reassert public service values of openness, probity and public accountability' operating within an ethical framework (NHS Management Executive, October 1993). The language of this circular suggests that somewhere along the way these values have been lost. Professionals adhere to their own established ethical frameworks, but as Wall, and then Cohen describe, these are constantly being confronted by those of the organisation in which they work, and they present fundamental problems of interpretation and meaning for both managers and professionals.

The traditional hierarchies are no longer fixed, but replaced by others that are constantly changing shape to meet external pressures, thus making it difficult to trace the past and relate it to the present. Professionals are now part of welfare institutions that have been systematically remade in a managerial mould, to fit a business entrepreneurial ideology. These new structures are created and sustained by the philosophical contention that individual freedom is linked to a market model of society organised on contractual relationships. But it must be remembered that these institutions are also founded on ideas of social justice, and if Douglas is right, it is they, as organisations, which 'make the big decisions', and these almost always involve ethical principles.

The NHS and social service departments have been deconstructed and reconstructed, placing professionals at the core – many in dual roles as managers and clinicians, both rationing and providing services on a face-to-face basis with clients and patients. But as well as consumer needs, the new services have to incorporate the needs and values of the individuals working within them, so that they can work efficiently. The 'Corporate Governance Strategy' will need to penetrate within the organisation and the minds of its professional members, referring to the past in order to formulate the present.

The challenge remains to find a congruence between the values of the professionals, and the objectives and ethical framework of the welfare institutions themselves. The government policy of the internal market at once seeks to depart from a past collectivist ideology and focus on an individualistic welfare market model free from the domination of professional groups, but at the same time there is a quest to maintain a collectivist stance, as the voices of Beveridge and Bevan are still echoing loudly from the past, and they live on in the public imagination. This difficult balancing act has to be achieved and sustained in order to continue to maintain the NHS as a universally freely accessible service. Returning to and bending Yeats's metaphorical language once more, the falcon must hear the falconer or else there is a danger that things may 'fall apart'.

References

Atkinson, P. (1983), 'The Reproduction of the Professional Community', in R. Dingwall and P. Lewis (eds), *The Sociology of the Professions* (London: Macmillan).

Beatham, D. (1987), *Bureaucracy* (Milton Keynes: Open University Press).

Becker, H. S., Geer, B., Hughes, E. L., and Strauss, A. L. (1960), *The Boys in White: Student Culture in Medical School* (Chicago: University of Chicago Press).

Bendix, R. (1977), *Max Weber: An Intellectual Portrait* (Cambridge: Cambridge University Press).

Blau, P. M. (1972), *The Dynamics of Bureaucracy* (Chicago: Phoenix Press).

Butler, J. and Calnan, M. (1988), *Too Many Patients? A study of the economy of time and standards of care in General Practice* (Aldershot: Avebury).

Chiplin, B. and Sloane, P. J. (1982), *Tackling Discrimination in the Workplace: An analysis of sex discrimination in Britain* (Cambridge: Cambridge University Press).

Cumberlege Report (1983), *Neighbourhood Nursing – A Focus for Care*, Report of the Community Nursing Review (London: HMSO).

Davies, C. (1983), 'Professionals in Bureaucracies: The conflict theory revisited', R. Dingwall and P. Lewis in (eds), *The Sociology of the Professions* (London: Macmillan).

Davies, C. and Rosser, J. (1986), *Processes of Discrimination: A study of women working in the NHS* (London: DHSS).

DHSS (1972), *Management Arrangements for the Reorganised National Health Service* (London: HMSO).

Douglas, M. (1987), *How Institutions Think* (London: Rouledge & Kegan Paul).

Drucker, P. (1979), *Management* (London: Pan Books).

Etzioni, A. (1969), *The Semi-Professions and their Organisations* (New York: Free Press).

Friedman, M. (1962), *Capitalism and Freedom* (Chicago: University of Chicago Press).

Game, A. and Pringle, R. (1983), *Gender at Work* (London: Pluto Press).

Garmarnikow, E. (1978), 'The Sexual Division of Labour: The case of nursing, in A. Kuhn and A. M. Wolpe (eds), *Feminism and Materialism* (London: Routledge & Kegan Paul).

Glennerster, H., Matsaganis, M., Owens, P. (1992), *A Foothold for Fundholding*, King's Fund Institute Research Report 12 (London: King's Fund).

Griffith's Report (1983), *Recommendations on the Effective Use of Manpower and Related Resources* (London: HMSO).

Klein, R. (1983), *The Politics of the National Health Service* (Harlow: Longman).

Kramer, R. M. (1981), *Voluntary Agencies in the Welfare State* (Berkeley: University of California Press).

Lévi-Strauss, C. (1977), *Structural Anthropology* (Harmondsworth: Penguin).

Malinowski, B. (1974), *Magic, Science and Religion and other Essays* (London: Souvenir Press).

Melia, K. (1987), *Learning and Working: The Occupational Socialization of Nurses* (London: Tavistock).

Mueller, D. (1979), *Public Choice* (Cambridge: Cambridge University Press).

NAHAT (1993–4), *NHS Handbook, 8th Edition* (Tunbridge Wells: JMH Publishing).

NHS Management Executive (1993) October Issue No 2 *Open to Account: Developments in Corporate Governance in the NHS* (Leeds: NHSME.)

Owens, P. and Glennerster, H. (1990), *Nursing in Conflict* (London: Macmillan).

Petch, H. and Owens, P. (1993), *The Bayswater Care Team; A Report for Kensington, Westminster and Chelsea Family Health Service Authority*, unpublished report by CAIPE, The London School of Economics.

Peters, T. S. and Waterman, R. H. (1982), *In Search of Excellence: Lessons from America's Best Run Companies* (New York: Harper & Row).

Salmon Report (1966), *Report on the Committee of Senior Nursing Staff Structure* (London: HMSO).

Salvage, J. (1985), *The Politics of Nursing* (London: Heinemann).

Scott, W. R. and Myer, J. W. (1983), *Organisational Environments: Ritual and Rationality* (London: Sage).

Strachey, L. (1918), *Eminent Victorians* (London: Chatto & Windus).

Titmuss, R. M. (1968), *Commitment to Welfare* (London: George Allen & Unwin).

UKCC (1986), *Project 2000: A New Preparation for Practice* (London: UK Central Council for Nursing, Midwifery and Health Visiting).

Weber, M. (1947), *The Theory of Social and Economic Organisation* (New York: Free Press).

3 Ethical and resource issues in health and social care

Andrew Wall

Chapter summary

This chapter addresses the theme of resource allocation and ethical judgements. It is on account of the dilemmas facing managers and doctors, constrained by limited budgets. Professional codes of conduct and financial imperatives may be in conflict and need resolution. The author focuses on managers and doctors specifically, as the two groups who have to prioritise services, make economic choices and address issues of equity. The tensions between utilitarian and individual philosophical approaches to resource allocation are at the heart of ethical debates. The author examines the complexities of meaning and perception that underlie these issues.

Stereotypical beliefs

Professionals, that is clinicians, working in health care are usually seen as ethically sound; managers, on the other hand, are viewed with suspicion. Social workers hold the middle ground. Clinicians are regulated by codes of conduct and infringement of these may result in a loss of the right to practise; managers face only the loss of their present job. In the health care setting there has yet to be an agreed code of conduct as to what managers should do and what is beyond the pale. This leads to considerable uneasiness among doctors, nurses and other clinicians who feel that economic pressures may interfere with their ability to treat their patient and this in turn will compromise their professional standards. All health systems are facing increasing financial difficulties and professionals are now being forced to face choices explicitly. Unfortunately, many of these professionals feel that managers are of little support in coping with these dilemmas and indeed, worse still, are entirely unsympathetic to anything but 'bottom line' financial outcomes.

But this crude depiction of the issue of ethical standards compromised by limited resources scarcely helps anyone and the stereotyping of the supposed conflict between clinicians, other caring professionals and managers is an abrogation of the need to face the fundamental issue that patients and clients and those that look after them cannot expect now or at any time that there will be unlimited resources at their disposal. Such a statement does not deny the need for ethical standards, rather it endorses them.

Ethical frameworks

But what are ethics? There is a danger that the word is used imprecisely in order to cast an air of respectability over loosely formulated principles which in more rigorous argument collapse. This chapter is not a philosophical essay, and therefore there will have to be some working description of what ethics are, which will allow issues to be explored without constantly returning to abstract and sometimes abstruse conceptual dialectic. Ethics are therefore described as being 'standards of conduct within the context of our social and economic systems'. The discussion will not be particularly concerned with what is often called 'medical ethics' and which usually ends up centering on euthanasia or birth control; the intention of this chapter, written by someone who is not a clinician but an erstwhile manager now working from an academic department largely with managers, is to examine rather more broadly the context of decision-making and how circumstances alter cases. The justification for this approach is a practical one: decisions have to be made, and if one person balks at some of the more difficult decisions, that only means someone else has to take on the task. It is therefore relevant to explore the credentials of those likely to be involved.

As already stated, professionals are regulated by codes of conduct supervised by accrediting bodies such as the General Medical Council (GMC), the Dental Practice Board, the United Kingdom Central Council for Nursing, Midwifery and Health Visiting (UKCC) and the Council for Professions Supplementary to Medicine. State registration is required and any alleged infringement of standards is examined with the prospect of a withdrawal of the right to practise if the professional is found to have acted improperly.

While this provides some safeguards for the public, it scarcely covers all eventualities. Professionals are therefore left with crucial decisions as to what to do in particular cases. Who should have what care at what cost is a fundamental issue facing all professionals any working day. The bodies who regulate them are not able to indicate, except in the most general terms, how professionals should set about making choices. Some professionals find choices which give to one and withhold from another unacceptable on the ground that such decisions betray their relationship with their patient or client. This is understandable and may well be where the manager, who does not have the same relationship with the patient, can be of use. The manager does not have an individual contract with the patient or client. But that does not mean that the manager is acting unethically; it signifies that the perspectives of manager and professional are different but equally valid.

This point needs some justification and perhaps the best way to do this is to explore the range of possible ethical frameworks within which professionals and managers alike make decisions. The NHS has often been depicted, along with the rest of the welfare state, as an example of utilitarian principles in action. Simply stated, that means that the welfare system aims to maximise benefits to the greatest number. Decisions in health care therefore will aim to improve health, to reduce suffering and to alleviate symptoms for the greatest number of people possible. Immediately the limitation of the utilitarian principle can be seen, in that such an approach could lead to some poor standards on the justification that everyone would get something, even if it was not very effective. The dangers go further, because by endorsing the mass benefits approach, there will be discrimination against those patients or clients who are chronically disabled, for whom a good result cannot be expected.

Utilitarianism and individualism

Managers tend to be depicted as being primarily influenced by the utilitarian view. Clinicians, are seen as being concerned only with the patient in front of them at any one time. Social workers are seen in a hybrid role – concerned for their clients - but with a greater recognition of the resource constraints. The prevailing professional view is that the patient's or client's rights are paramount and that the cost consequences are of secondary importance. The public seem to take the same view. Recent examples of the cost of treating children needing transplant surgery suggest that the public readily accept that providing health care should somehow be above mundane considerations of cost; in other words the rights of the individual are supreme. As potential individual patients, we would all hope that, when we have need for treatment, our clinicians and our managers will take the view that everything possible should be done. Similarly, protecting the rights of children has often involved social services departments in very high levels of expenditure which managers would be brave to challenge too publicly.

That of course is the crux of the matter – everything *possible* should be done. Do we mean clinically, socially or financially? Most clinicians will expect that their clinical judgements will have to be checked against resources. But this may lead to pragmatism, and for many people ethics is about absolute principles which cannot be compromised by circumstance. So, for instance, clinicians will maintain that the patient has the right to confidentiality, even where the courts may ask for information to be revealed. In fact, this absolutist position cannot easily be upheld. If the protection of a child requires the sharing of information between clinicians, other professional workers and even on occasions concerned voluntary staff, it would be an obtuse person who refused to share what they know which could improve the management of the case.

Some clinical staff feel that the discussion of ethics becomes too academic in all events and that their duty is more simply expressed as a duty to care, acting altruistically in their patients's interests (McFarlane, 1988); the doing is what is required. But this view is limiting and no help at all when issues regarding the distribution of resources are under discussion.

Last, in this review of ethical frameworks, is the attempt to decide what to do by testing the patient's own eligibility, the ethics of just desserts. Within this approach decisions are made in favour of the most worthy: so the virtuous receive, those who are considered reprehensible do not. Before professionals scoff at the unlikelihood of this approach prevailing, it is worth recalling the recent discussion on the priority downgrading of smokers for cardiac surgery or of the challenge to the right of an unmarried woman to receive infertility treatment. In both highly publicised instances opinions were expressed which were motivated by the belief that the patient was in some way unworthy – even guilty – and therefore ineligible for treatment. In social work such a process of thinking can wreck relationships with clients. In both health and social services settings, the result is discrimination of a most troubling kind. Nevertheless, the approach cannot entirely be ignored if the ground shifts slightly towards considering the consequences of choosing patients for treatment who may prove to be poor risks or who may be expensive to care for in the long term.

Painful choices

What this discussion has endeavoured to point out is that no one ethical standpoint will hold good in all circumstances and this is true for clinicians, other professionals and for managers equally (Wall, 1993). For many people this is unsatisfactory. If every decision is merely a rehearsal of points of view, how are patients, clients, the public and professionals themselves to be assured that the right things are being done? And, more particularly, can the suspicion that in the end managers make the crucial decisions as to how resources are to be used be allayed? Obviously not. The need for managers in one sense can be justified on the ground that, if practitioners were able to make up their own minds, managers would not be required. Managers have increasingly been brought into organisations just because others could not make decisions because of the complexity of the issues facing them. Whereas it is a relatively simple matter to decide on a simple treatment for a patient with a well-understood set of symptoms, or a client with a single social need, it becomes much more difficult to judge the appropriate distribution of resources across a community.

The differences between doctors and other health professionals and managers are often stressed. At one level the discussion is not so much about the ethics surrounding choices but more a simple challenge for power. In the ethical debate this is unhelpful as neither party can convincingly claim either to have moral superiority or to be in the best place to exert it. It is more helpful to examine the respective roles of clinical staff *vis-à-vis* managers and in so doing to demonstrate that both have legitimacy and both need to be able to demonstrate an ethical approach to their tasks. One way of showing this is to take a look at the continuum of care and endeavour to find the decision points along that line.

A patient cannot be so named until he or she has seen a doctor or health professional of similar status. This is important because the patient is only legitimised by this giving of a name: without the title he or she cannot proceed along the continuum of care. So we may call this *the point of legitimisation*. Once named 'patient', the person is eligible for the use of resources. These are commanded by the clinician working on the patient's behalf but ultimately the resources stem from management, so we call this point along the continuum *the point of authorisation*. Further along still, we arrive at *the point of satisfaction* when the patient confirms explicitly or, more likely, implicitly by responding to treatment, their satisfaction with the process (providing, of course, that they are satisfied).

The purpose of this sort of model is that it first centres on the patient and his or her needs and secondly it removes images of conflict and polarity from the discussion of the roles of clinical and managerial staff. In this model the parties are contracted to the same task of trying to meet the patient's needs. The model can be rejected, of course, on the grounds that it only works with those people who are seeking patient status; what about the greater health needs of the community in general? What about the potential conflict between medical and social models of care? Here indeed we do have other dilemmas. In health care settings, however much politicians, academics and managers postulate the need to create a healthier community through the means of health promotion, the resources set aside for this objective are small. Of course we would all like to see a healthier society, but the fact is that most decisions about health care are about how to manage sickness. Similarly, and at the risk of making heretical statements, the 'shift' to the community from secondary institutional care is stronger on rhetoric than on achievement. This is not cynical, merely a recognition of the facts, at least to date.

Questions of power

The discussion so far has centred on the roles of those who have to make key decisions on the patients' behalf. It has been suggested that the traditional adversarial model of professionals versus managers is unhelpful in dealing with this unenviable task of deciding priorities. But professionals may still feel that they are being compromised by some of the decisions which have to be made.

Many professionals feel that they now have a greater problem in looking after their patients and clients because of the increased interference by government in the process and the ever growing power of managers (at least in the NHS), particularly in the last ten years since the advent of general management. Local government has lost power during the same period and there is now, in any case, a considerable imbalance between managers in the NHS and their counterparts in social services departments. This leads to considerable problems when they are negotiating common solutions. But at the same time there has also been a renewed and more determined attempt to involve clinicians in decision-making. Clinical management is now a major issue and this means that the importance of the relationship between input of resources and the outcome of effective care and treatment is more explicitly acknowledged. A report (Dixon, 1990) emphasises the importance of the clinical directorate system led by doctors. There is therefore a recognition that clinicians need to bridge what they themselves have in the past seen as a chasm between what the patient needs ideally and what in practical terms they are likely to get.

Should professionals feel compromised by this recognition of reality? Some commentators would maintain that doctors have taken too much of the ethical high ground in the past and have therefore only themselves to blame when they find they cannot continue to defend it all. A good doctor, this argument suggests, knows the limits of his or her practice, and that clinical intervention is not always what is required (Seedhouse, 1991). But the problem is whether or not the public or the doctor's own patient are willing for the doctor to admit these limitations. As Halper puts it:

> Is the physician left with an unresolvable conflict of interest, ostensibly pursuing the patient's best interest but often feeling compelled to place a societal interest in efficient resource allocation first? (1989, p. 152)

The answer must presumably be that the conflict is not unresolvable, but it is difficult. Given the team setting in which many decisions regarding patients are made, the assumption of the prime role of the doctor in this process may increasingly be challenged. But how should all involved behave?

Principles of action

The first principle, and that most commonly referred to, is the one which recognises autonomy, both that appertaining to the patient and that to his or her clinician. Other principles are an obligation to do the best your skills have equipped you to do for your patient; the obligation not knowingly to do harm to your patient; and a commitment to justice which may cover, at one level, whistleblowing when things are perceived as going wrong or at another level – and more fundamentally – endeavouring to achieve equity for patients and clients and, more widely, the whole community.

Let us examine each of these in a little more detail. The principle of autonomy can lead to conflict in that respecting the patient's point of view may challenge the tendency towards paternalism which is implicit in every clinician–patient relationship. Simply, the patient wants the doctor to make them better. Yet it is also true that the patient wishes to have his or her individuality respected, to be treated like a person rather than a case and to be empowered, at least a little, in order to be able to manage their illness or disability in the longer term. The principle therefore honours respect more than it sanctifies uniqueness of the patient (Brecher 1988, p. 42; Harris, 1992, p. 200).

What happens to this principle when applied to doctors themselves? At the bottom of many of the discussions of clinical autonomy is the traditional battle by a professional group to seek independence to practise unrestrained by the government of the day or their servants, in this case NHS managers. Some scepticism is therefore justified if it is maintained that come what may, the doctor must have his way on behalf of his patient.

Doctors, of course, are accountable. First they are accountable to their patients, and despite the regressive instincts of many patients under treatment, are expected to explain the nature of their decisions regarding the patient in front of them. Secondly, doctors are also accountable to the organisation more generally. This is sometimes contested on the basis that professions exist outside the context of the current management. This elitist view, understandable though it may be coming from a highly skilled body of people, is nevertheless inadmissible in ethical terms. The skills that doctors acquire come from their education which, at least in the UK, will have been publically funded. A duty therefore exists to pay back to society what society so readily sponsors in the first place.

It is helpful to recall the elements of clinical autonomy. First there is the right to independent practice allowed by the system and regulated by a body recognised by government and the judiciary. Secondly, autonomy is recognised by the right of the patient to choose a clinician and the clinician to choose the patient. This right can of course be abused on both sides and some clinicians will be sorely tempted to rid themselves of patients whom they find difficult in some way. Ethically they have to ask themselves whether the interests of the patient can be maintained if the doctor acts in this way.

Another crucial element of autonomy as described by Jaques and colleagues in their seminal work on health service organisation

(Jaques *et al.*, 1978) is the concept of prime responsibility, whereby one clinician accepts the role of looking after the patient's interests even though a team of people may be involved. Subtly different is the principle of primacy which maintains that prime responsibility in health care falls *first* to the doctor. Autonomy therefore is a concept which does not automatically ensure ethical behaviour from clinicians; there are too many challenges to allow that to be said. Nevertheless discussion of the issues goes some way to providing an ethical framework within which the relationship of patient to clinician can be managed.

The next principle which may help is that which requires the clinician to do the best he or she can for the patient. If they do that, the argument goes, they will be acting ethically. The drawback is the question as to how far the clinician is expected to influence the resources which might be available to his or her patient. Is the clinician to expect others to make the macro allocation of resources and accept that his or her role is limited to the day-to-day decisions as to the allocating of the budget? Clinical directors largely work on that principle and it is on the whole reasonable. But on the other hand, only clinicians know at first hand what their patients can best benefit from, and it must be expected that clinicians will act as advocates in their patient's interests and will not therefore be inclined to accept the status quo. So there are judgments to be made as to what 'doing your best' really means.

Complementary to the principle of doing your best is not knowingly doing harm. In clinical terms this is rather harder to honour than might first appear. There are numerous procedures, treatments and medications which are in themselves unpleasant for the patient. At what point does unpleasantness degenerate into harm? There are other instances where the clinician is not aware of the harm until much later. Is he or she to be considered guilty of ethical turpitude because they have engaged in a course of treatment for their patient without knowing all the possible consequences of that action? An explicit assessment of consequences will help to demonstrate that the clinician is acting ethically.

Managers are not exposed to such a rigorous process: seldom do they have to demonstrate that they have acted ethically. In some ways less is expected of them. They do not have any claim to autonomy – only to power, and that is different. They may feel that in a general way they are there to do their best, and managers in the public service may still espouse the public service ethos. Obviously they would not wish to be seen as doing anyone harm, but all too

numerous examples exist where employees have clearly suffered at
the hands of their managerial superiors.

The issue of equity

The ethical worlds of clinicians and managers are often different but
in some ways overlap, particularly in the area of the principle of
justice. At a macro level managers, with clinical colleagues and with
public health specialists, are much concerned with interpreting the
principle of equity within health services. Everyone would broadly
support the view that the distribution of resources should be fair. But
that one word is not as simple as it looks, because there are various
ways in which fairness can be demonstrated.

Does it mean that all potential patients with similar conditions
should have equal access to services? Or alternatively, does it mean
that only patients with similar conditions should have equal access,
on the grounds that it is pointless to compare the access of a road
accident patient with someone awaiting a hip replacement or a
mother in labour with a man with chronic bronchitis? Should access
be determined by the ability of the patient to benefit or, returning to
arguments stated above, because the patient has the right to care and
treatment irrespective of the level of benefit he or she is likely to
derive from it? Is fairness to be interpreted as an opportunity to
receive equal shares or, alternatively, to receive unequal shares
determined by need? This is not the place to fillet these arguments in
detail; it is enough to demonstrate that equity as a principle is
difficult to handle.

Crudely speaking, the NHS endeavours to allocate resources according to need, but there are numerous examples where other
pressures have subverted that principle. Clinicians act as advocates
for their patients and, in the last resort, may have to leave the
final decisions to managers and to the boards of management they in
turn serve. But there remains a feeling of discomforture that there
are no cast-iron ethical arguments to resolve some of these dilemmas.

Because of this unease, some staff feel the need to expose the issue
to view especially when they feel that the public are being kept in
the dark. 'Whistleblowing', as it has come to be called, has become
such an issue that at least one of the professional bodies has found it
necessary to issue guidance (RCN, 1992). The justification for this is
an attempt to make things better. What the guidance symbolises is a

more responsive management process, leading to higher morale amongst staff and greater satisfaction amongst patients.

Whose values?

What this discussion on ethics has also demonstrated is that professionals are in the end guided by their own set of values. Rules are inadequate, sanctions are insufficient, to ensure that conduct will be always be at the highest standard. But this is also a minefield. Whose values are to be blessed, whose to be condemned and by whom?

An exercise conducted by the author during discussion on ethics with a wide range of health staff, clinical and managerial, has demonstrated that instinctively judgements are made about who should be treated first from a basis of who in society is more worthy. The result was the same with doctors as with managers, in that a 35-year-old male patient with three children requiring renal transplant was seen as more deserving than a 20-year-old single woman requiring the same procedure and certainly more so than a man or a women of 75 requiring hip replacement. The reasons given were social: 'he has dependents', and economic: 'he has years of productive work ahead of him'. These views were then put under pressure by revealing that the man has never worked and that his family, all three children by different mothers, was entirely supported by state benefits. The discussion ended in confusion, but not before it had demonstrated how automatic are some of our responses even among those whose professional training might have led them to be more wary before making such choices.

Professionals need to be aware that decisions are made in a variety of different modes. It is reasonable to assume that a professional will make a rational decision, which in health choices means that the outcomes have been carefully estimated and that an equation has been struck between benefit and cost. But equally we can demonstrate that decisions are also reached in other modes. Children are flown in from the battlefront because politicians and newspapermen wish to take credit, to influence world affairs and to satisfy the emotions of their respective electorates and readers. Cooler counsels prevail when professionals and managers get together and decide through the process of consensus.

This has considerable potential in tackling some of the larger priority debates in the health service today. Some philosophers have argued that it is in vain that we try to make the right decisions about resource allocation as every argument can be challenged. Instead, random allocation might well be as fair. The problem is that in the minds of people generally it is just unacceptable to expose themselves and their loved ones to a lottery, 'fair' or not.

Professionals have an unenviable task. They are expected to exemplify the principle that they have the interests of their patients at heart, uncompromised by consideration of resources. But, as has been argued, such a position is untenable: not only because it is unrealistic but also because it is not in the end more ethical than a position which accepts that choices have to be made in the context of resources. This dilemma has affected professionals who have decided to exert their professional freedom. The word liberty is often used at this stage as a last attempt to safeguard the rights of the individual, whether patient or clinician. But it proves fruitless on the basis that my freedom is usually only bought at your expense: if I have, you may not.

Working together

So how can professionals working in health services be best advised? To begin with, there needs to be a commitment to mutual respect. Clearly this encompasses a respect for the patient but it also needs to acknowledge the contribution made by managers and professionals alike. This is not necessarily easy, given the different degrees of independence of each profession: emerged, emerging, or not-yet-emerged from medical domination. An interesting example of the caterpillar into butterfly is the suggestion that other professionals are now ready to become equal partners in general practice. This in turn puts pressure on the principle of primary responsibility referred to above. Clinical psychologists will be well used to negotiating their status in mental health settings, as will be social workers ready to challenge medical domination, from an allied but different bureaucracy.

Secondly, despite some reservations (Hunter, 1993), there is increasing support for decisions about health care resources being made more explicit. It is argued that in a sophisticated society there can be little justification for keeping many of these fundamental discussions about resources and professional interventions under wraps. Just because the discussion is difficult is no reason for not having in public. How else are patients to appreciate the problems and to grow in their ability to handle these fundamental human dilemmas as to who shall get what in health care?

With mutual respect and a greater openness there might emerge a greater acceptance that professionals, like managers, now need to acknowledge that they work not only *in* a state-run system (however fragmented it becomes) but that they also work *for* it, for a common single purpose.

References

Brecher, B. (1988), in Fairburn G. and Fairburn S. (eds), *Ethical Issues in Caring* (Aldershot: Avebury).

Dixon, M. (1990), *Models of Clinical Management* (London: Institute of Health Services Management).

Halper, T. (1989), *The Misfortunes of Others* (Cambridge: Cambridge University Press).

Harris, J. (1992), *The Value of Life* (London: Routledge).

Hunter, D. (1993), *Rationing Dilemmas in Health Care*, Research Paper No.8 (Birmingham: NAHAT).

Jaques, E. ed. (1978), *Health Services* (London: Heinemann).

McFarlane, J. (1988), 'Nursing: a paradigm for caring', in G. Fairburn and S. Fairburn (ed), *Ethical Issues in Caring* (Aldershot: Avebury).

RCN (1992), *Whistleblow*, a report (London: RCN).

Seedhouse, D. (1991), *Liberating Medicine* (Chichester: Wiley).

Wall, A. (1993), *Values and the NHS* (London: Institute of Health Services Management).

4 *The market and professional frameworks*

Anna Cohen

Chapter summary

This chapter develops the themes, outlined in Chapter 3, of resource allocation and service development. The author draws on her own anthropological study to explore the world of the internal market, and the new concepts of contract and competition in the NHS. The study illustrates the divergent perspectives of managers and clinicians in the decision-making context, and the linguistic barriers that exist and which prevent achievement of mutual understanding and commonly agreed objectives. The powerful role of the purchasers in defining health and social care presents new challenges to front-line professionals providing care.

Contracts and purchasers

In this chapter I want to look at some of the problems raised by the changes in the organisational and legal framework of the health service. I shall focus on how the change to an internal market system implies a new way of thinking about health care and new relationships between clinicians and managers; and I analyse how the various professional groups have responded to the change and how their conflicting attitudes influence the way they work together. In particular I want to examine certain key concepts – such as the purchaser–provider split, 'contract', needs assessment and priority-setting – which arise in both the health sector and in community care, to explore both the way in which different professional groups interpret them and the resulting patterns of communication. The changes are not straightforward and the conflicting models of health care held by different professional groups have tended to increase ambiguity over areas of responsibility and decision-taking rather than clarity as intended.

The findings are drawn from research carried out in one Health Authority over a three-year period, from shortly before the introduction of the health service reform in April 1991 until the end of 1993. Information was obtained through observation of meetings between professionals in various fora and through interviews. The data used derive from both hospital and community units, but it is intended that the points made should have a more general relevance, as the same model is applied in social services as well as health care.

The 1991 NHS reform

Until 1991 the NHS functioned according to a relatively simple model. In a pyramidal hierarchical structure, policy and control flowed down from government via the Department of Health to increasingly smaller geographical and organisational entities – Regions, Districts and finally hospital and community units (Klein, 1983). Resources passed down through the system in the same way, ending up allocated to the hospital and community units (Harrison *et al.*, 1990). Under the new system, the health service is re-structured to conform more closely to the model of enterprise in the private sector (Harden, 1992). Districts and GP fundholders are now to act as purchasers of health care, on behalf of their local populations and practice patients, from hospital and community units which act as providers of health services. Money is held by the purchaser to buy health care and the arrangements for purchasing are spelled out in 'contracts' or 'service agreements'. The 'contract' consists of a description of the service to be purchased, the quality of care to be provided, the number of interventions to be made, the monitoring of the 'contract' through the collection of information and follow-up procedures, the cost or price of the total number of interventions made and finally standard terms covering dispute resolution and failure to meet terms. Implicit in the reorganisation is a change in role. The purchaser is to be responsible for finding out the health needs of the population and buying appropriate services, whilst the provider is to be concerned only with the running of the service.

Whilst much of the reform is organisational and financial, other themes play a part in the motivation for change as stated in the legislation. It is intended that the move to a more private sector approach will lead to increased choice for the patient over where and when health care is received and that such choices, expressed through GPs and particularly GP fund holders, will lead to competition between provider units to offer services of appropriate or better quality in a more cost-effective way. That is, the reform is intended to emphasise the rights of the patient and to lead to quality and efficiency gains.

The next section explores some of the hidden assumptions in the market model and the extent to which it can usefully be applied to the provision of health care (a similar point is made by Hughes, who contrasts the usual meaning of key concepts such as 'contract' and 'trust' in the private sector with their restricted scope in the NHS [Hughes, 1991]).

The market model

One of the dominant discourses of our culture is that of the market – the efficient and best allocation of resources through the meeting of supply and demand. In addition, it contains an idea of the individual as someone able to determine her or his own life, a subject freed from relationships, context, and history. Finally, a third element is that of the role of government, which is to withdraw from most areas of personal life and leave the individual free to choose how to live and the market to operate most effectively. Implicit in the NHS reform then, is a particular view of public services. This lies in the contrast drawn between the market and the public sector and it is this which makes the contemporary market model new and different from those of the past. Public services, in this view, are assumed to be and are presented as wasteful, bureaucratic and as reflecting the interests of particular professional groups rather than of those they theoretically serve. All this is undoubtedly true in part. But it is important to focus on those strands of the health service reform which express an ideological construct rather than the technical transformation of health care. In fact, it is this image of the reform as simply a technical transformation which tends to throw up problems for professionals of all sorts working in health care, since it acts to obscure or silence debate over issues which professionals find ethically or practically difficult to resolve.

The market then is presented as a neutral and more efficient way of allocating resources because the process is removed from personal, irrational choices and power. It is therefore thought to be fairer and to transfer power from professional elites to the service-user. The flow of resources and statements of quality are formally codified in 'contracts', that is, they are brought out into the light of day and can be monitored. In this model, the manager, whether purchaser, provider or GP fund holder, becomes the representative and advocate of the patient.

In evaluating the effectiveness of the NHS reform, it is necessary to consider to what degree a rational, open system based on market forces has replaced personal and local considerations. The model builds on a positivist view of reality; that is, that social reality is like physical reality, with laws that can be laid bare by using scientific methods of various sorts and that, in turn, it can be altered and manipulated in a straightforward way.

An alternative view of reality is put forward by the anthropologist Clifford Geertz who argues that our perception and understanding of the world is shaped by the culture we live in: 'man is an animal suspended in webs of significance he himself has spun' (Geertz, 1973, p. 5). Writers as diverse as Weber (1976), Gramsci (1971) and Foucault (1963) have explored the different world-views held by social groups and the process by which the interests of one group, and their version of reality, come to dominate and replace the others (Foucault, 1963; Gramsci, 1971; Weber, 1976). In other words, where the health service reform assumes that all is straightforward and simple, the reality is rather of the co-existence of different professional groups (not to mention patients and the lay population), each with contrasting attitudes to illness and health and expectations about medicine and the market.

Medicine itself as a practice is historically constructed. The NHS is inextricably a technical, political and ethical institution, both practical and symbolic. Within it the practice of medicine and relationships between patients and doctors, nurses and other paramedics reflects the shifting authority of medical elites within society at different periods of time. The meaning of illness, emotions and the body is shaped by entry into a ritualised domain constructed by medical and nursing knowledge, in which the person becomes a patient and which provides an interpretation or understanding of health and illness, death, the emotional and the personal. Medicine then, is one of the ways in which we understand our experience, it shapes it for us, and the doctor and nurse are charismatic figures (Lakoff and Johnson, 1980). In the popular perception it is a domain very different from that of the market.

The following section explores the way in which these two models – that of medicine and that of the market – interact as professionals attempt to introduce the reforms. I shall argue that the reform implies a new construction of illness; of the patient – doctor – nurse relationship; and of the ethical basis on which health care resources are allocated. Words and symbols transported from the private sector, in Burke's terms, cluster together, constituting the central way in which reality is to be perceived and ordered afresh (Burke, 1969). The key criteria of action are efficiency, accountability, devolved responsibility; changes are validated by endless comparisons with Sainsbury's, Marks & Spencer, ICI; medical practices are renamed, specialities become service delivery units, consultants are clinical directors, patients are consumers. Health service time begins anew with the creation of a chronology starting from 'year one' of the market.

Yet the market model is a very specific one and in many ways it may be unable to resolve the difficulties currently facing the health service – those related to decisions over how resources are to be allocated. A startling ambiguity lies at the heart of the NHS internal market. In the private sector, according to the classical law of contract, a contract is an agreement made between two parties to exchange goods or services for money. In the case of default either party can go to law. But in the NHS reform the legislation rules out resort to the law courts. What status then do NHS 'contracts' have? Are they binding or not? If not, why go to the trouble of writing them at all? Such issues preoccupied professionals and generated many conflicts. Again, a market model envisages only consumers and purchasers who interact on the basis of demand. Yet health care, if it is to be equitable and effective requires that those who are without power are taken into consideration in the planning of a full range of services, and that the public interest is central – and this may run counter to the efficient working of the market. However, before turning to a closer discussion of this kind of issue I want to examine how the reform has been interpreted by various groups of professionals, and explore the way in which first, managers, and then clinicians and nurses, construct their professional identities.

The managers

Managers, whether District purchasers or hospital or community unit providers often appear superficially to be open to the reform. As we shall see, they interpret the implications of the market in different ways.

The reform is largely one which redefines the managerial role and power. In the view of managers the health service has historically been dominated by consultants, in which allocation of resources has depended on who shouts loudest and on 'horse- trading'. However, GPs have always determined the pattern of referrals, their significance has only fully come to be appreciated by managers with the advent of the reform and, in particular, the introduction of GP fundholders.

In this construction of the health service – which rings true – managers have related to a group of largely autonomous consultants in their separate specialties who have all been jockeying for scarce resources. The power of the manager or administrator, and at the same time what they perceive as their weakness, was essentially 'feudal' in this account – they rewarded those who did favours for them, or the most powerful. They essentially steered between the rivals, playing a mediating, consensus role, negatively seen as 'centralist' or 'despotic' as they sought to control spending (Strong and Robinson, 1990).

For the purchasers, the legislation offers an opportunity to gain power at last over the consultants who have throughout the history of the NHS largely determined its shape. Thus a purchaser talks about needs assessment in the following way:

> It's all provider driven at the moment because we're in the hands of providers and they're encouraging us to say 'leave it in our hands, dear'. [But] the group that chose these areas [for needs assessment] was looking at how we can make rational decisions and use money different-ly. (Director of Nursing Services)

Purchasers see the existing pattern of health care delivery as chaotic, the outcome of pressure by the most powerful consultants and specialities and uncontrolled expenditure by individual doctors and specialities which fails to meet the needs of the population. There are two slightly different perspectives here. One focuses on the market as offering the chance to make consultants responsible for their use of resources and therefore more careful – this is through the setting up of service delivery units, as they are called, with their own budgets, and which will manage themselves. The other view sees the market as offering the chance for management to become more controlling as purchasers decide what health care to buy. They see this as a more 'rational', 'scientific', 'explicit' system of resource allocation compared with the old-style 'slopping around' and 'fudging', and say :

> The real benefits . . . are making choices between priorities explicit and trying to make those choices on basis of population need. (Director of Purchasing)

The objectives . . . are about satisfying patients rather more, satisfying their needs etc. etc. but inevitably funding for the NHS is not a bottom-less pit so we can only attempt to satisfy these various needs within certain levels of resources. (Finance Director – Trust Hospital)

The purpose of the reforms should be about trying to get money to follow patients where they actually need services . . . about using your resources in the best and most effective way . . . It should mean that you should be able to treat more people within the same resources or you should be able to make service shifts so you move resources and ration your resources in a way that makes the best fit. (Assistant Director of Finance, Purchasing)

For managers of provider hospital and community units who have to be responsible for preventing individual specialties over-spend-ing:

Our aim as a hospital and the aim of the Unit management . . . is to strengthen the management of our clinical teams . . . so they identify them-selves as a team managing their service, rather than the team just practising their medicine. (Deputy Unit General Manager)

Purchasers and unit managers think the reform will lead to alter-ations in clinical practice as doctors and nurses begin to be respon-sible for managing their own speciality budgets and become conscious of the relation between resources and treatment:

Doctors are used to taking clinical decisions based on their medical judgement but if they commit money . . . to one group of patients it is being denied to another . . . they . . . have to make a decision about what they do and what they don't do. (Deputy Unit General Manager)

Such changes are viewed both positively and negatively. In the long term, some believe, the reform might lead to a re-think of the purpose and function of the NHS and the replacement of the tradi-tional individual patient-orientated approach of clinicians with that of a process of rational assessment. Such a shift would give managers more power within the health service as they become the repre-sentatives of the whole group of patients whose needs and treatment they attempt to balance in an overt way:

> The health service has always been log-jammed by money. One of the benefits – some of you might say it is not – of contracting is that you have an explicit statement of what you are going to buy. Most of those people waiting [for treatment] are not in a life-threatening position. What is the NHS for? Is it to do with life-threatening circumstances . . . or is it meant to be for the varicose veins? (Unit Finance Director)

This unit finance director criticises surgeons who always opt to treat the most sick patient and, in making these decisions, 'play God'. Rather there should be an assessment of the patient: looking at the success of the procedure, life-expectancy, and quality of life. (In later sections I shall explore some of the difficulties implicit in introducing this approach.) For all managers a further benefit of the reform is that:

> It has loosened up the old bureaucratic structure – District and Region breathing down your neck the whole time . . . [with] nothing better to do than faxing out forms to be filled in . . . You think why on earth do they want this, who is running this hospital, them or us?   (Unit Finance Director)

The NHS is described as 'over-bureaucratic', with 'the mentality of the civil service and an organisation set up during the Second World War' (Deputy Unit General Manager, Trust hospital). Managers were locked in rivalries between Units, between Units and District, and with the rest of the NHS hierarchy. The object – and this is equally true for the other groups in the system – is to appear to do what 'our masters' have told us but to obtain scarce resources. In this there is a clear demarcation of knowledge so that Region will be portrayed by District as out of touch, motivated by political needs, bureaucratic in much the same way as Units see District. Rhetoric and images are consciously manipulated in order to control other players so that great attention is paid to words.

Professional groups tend to act strategically with an eye to manipulating other groups or concealing their practice from them. Many managers are highly critical of the Department of Health, for its bureaucracy and distance from the realities of the health service, and of politicians in general for their short-term political interests which convert the NHS into a 'political football' and frequently, if not always, run against the interests of patients. This means, very significantly, that managers as a whole tend to be using the reform as an opportunity to introduce the changes they feel are necessary and to distinguish themselves from the political objectives:

> The bottom line original objective of the reforms was just . . . to find a way of tackling the cash crisis in the NHS, at least from a political point of view . . . The line here has been . . . that reforms offered us an opportunity to improve local services and improve services to local residents in new ways and we were going to seize those opportunities in ways that we felt best locally. We weren't going to follow national and regional guidance to the last letter.   (Director of Purchasing)

To summarise these complex points of view, managers see themselves as operating in a largely chaotic and hierarchical system in which they try to introduce a rational, scientific approach but are aware of their own weakness to achieve this goal. They see themselves as the representative of the patient but their objectives are defined in relation to a generalised mass of potential patients. This contrasts very strongly with the view of clinicians.

The doctors and nurses

In contrast to the managerial representation of identity and responsibility is that of clinicians – doctors, nurses and paramedics – and their construction of the doctor–nurse–patient role. They too see themselves as the representative of the patient, but in their vision of themselves they are the ones who provide the service:

> I don't mean that people working at District or at Unit level don't see the end point as being patient care. But because they don't have the exposure to the patients directly or their families – that isn't such an acute feeling for them. You might argue that it's important that it isn't so that they can stand back and be objective – I won't say dispassionate . . . (Consultant)

They are caring and concerned, involved in a concrete way with the patient, and unlike the management, talk about the reality of illness and dying. This is a very powerful self-image and it underpins the reluctance – particularly of consultants – to become involved in what they see as 'administration'. Clinicians base their viewpoint on what they see as their closer knowledge of the situation; they have a different perspective on what the problems of the health service are. For example, where disagreement had arisen between purchasers and the clinical team over the number of cases seen in the previous year:

> We just know that is totally wrong . . . we know what we have on the ward . . . and if official figures don't match, then ours were obviously right. (Senior Nurse)

> In relation to paediatric cardiology we had extremely accurate data . . . those data was ignored in the production of contracts . . . I found it frustrating that people seemed adamant that they were going to use data that we knew were inaccurate. (Consultant)

This constitutes a critique of the reform:

> For years District haven't given us enough money to be able to deliver the service as well as we would be able to. It's now just put in slightly different terms . . . however you re-arrange it if there isn't enough money to give you're going to end up with the same problem. So it's now in a contract – I mean a piece of paper . . . we've just slightly re-arranged the ways an inadequate sum of money is handed on to us to fulfil the needs of the children who come to us. (Consultant)

With reference to the process of needs assessment being carried out by purchasers:

> All that has been done is people have gone to individual departments and asked how many patients were treated last year, the waiting list . . . is there other information than that? . . . I think there is a lot of talk and a lot of work basically is management, business management coming in and terminology . . . but no extra information behind it . . .   (Consultant)

Their construction of medicine is concerned with the provision of care to individual patients on the basis of need and some clinicians contrast this ethic sharply with that of managers whom they term – significantly – 'administrators':

> The health service is about individuals, it's about providing medical services for individuals and this is provided normally by professionals well-trained who have dedicated their lives to this. Management is not in the least concerned about providing medical services to individual patients . . . often . . . is not dedicated to the health service . . . is em-

ployed for their managerial abilities, that is to say, to balance the books. (Consultant)

> Businessmen are liars and engage in chicanery – you do this not just to earn a living but because you want to help people a bit. People have to have trust, confidence in you – the doctor . . . That's how they see us as people who know a lot and help. (Consultant)

There is a clear sense of contrasting ethics:

> I think we need better figures and I think it probably will help to define the service but I don't think you can turn away sick children . . . I really feel if people are ill they should be treated and I cannot reconcile the ethical economy resource issues, I find that very difficult. I don't think it is wrong to think about costs but I don't really and truly believe in this market. The whole point of business is to make money, there is no other point whatsoever and that is not the health care business, is it? (Senior Nurse)

The next section examines how, in trying to implement the new system, the two approaches – that of managers and that of clinicians – clashed. To some extent this reflected a problem of communication: if different words had been used, there might have been greater agreement over how to resolve difficulties. But it is also true that the two professional groups have different kinds of experience and knowledge which are not shared and that each seeks to impose its own definition of the problems and their resolution on the situation. To these fundamental disparities is added the ambiguity and incoherence generated by the market model itself, and the inability of those trying to apply it to resolve problems by means of it.

In three areas of the reform ambiguity arises, and the two contrasting approaches and identities of managers and clinicians emerge clearly, resulting in irresolvable dilemmas and deadlock in decision-making.

Conflicting paradigms

Competition and 'contract'

As discussed earlier, in the market model a contract is a legally binding document with resort to penalties. The NHS 'contract' however is a very ambiguous concept, although it is a crucial plank in the health service reforms, along with the idea of competition. In describing how professionals coped with introducing and creating 'contracts' for services, we are led into their fundamental feelings and attitudes towards the reform in general. The making of 'contracts' was not a straightforward process governed by such factors as quality and cost, but a very complex one shaped by the hidden context of different approaches and professional identities, contrasting interpretations and objectives, and both professional and personal strategies. In addition the making of 'contracts' was characterised by uncertainties and ambiguities over the accuracy of information, the status of the agreement (was it binding or not?), and finally over the setting of the price.

Providers were not allowed to set their own prices but could only charge as much for a service as they had received for it in the past, plus inflation. Hence, the great focus on getting the workload figures right. If the number of interventions laid down in the 'contract' did not reflect the number of interventions made or requested or needed during the following year, there would be inadequate resources available. Meetings between purchasers and providers to establish a 'contract' were often conflictual as professionals sought to shape the agreement to meet their definition of what happened in that particular part of the service, what was wrong with it in their view and what was needed. On the clinical side, nurses often had different agendas from those of doctors, whilst in turn unit management had concerns which differed from those of purchasing managers and again from clinicians. Such differences were reflected in practice as each group adopted a different strategy not only towards the 'contract', but also to the process of negotiation.

Nurses' concerns tended to be to ensure that the 'contract' contained a clear description of nursing practice with an emphasis on its increasing professionalism, nurse education and changing practice in relation to the patient. This was a movement away from seeing the patient only as a medical case to a more holistic approach focusing on the patient's needs for care both within the hospital and outside, and on the social context of the patient's life. In addition they were anxious to ensure that the need for highly specialised nurses was made clear, as this tended to increase the quality of the service at the expense of a greater cost or price and they did not want this to be questioned. Finally, in specialities which were hard pressed for resources nurses were keen to have the problems this entailed for a high quality service spelled out in special 'areas of concern' sections of the 'contract'. It is clear that nurses as a professional group had both patient-orientated and interest group concerns in relation to the description of the service and that they perceived the 'contract' as important, with consequences for resources, professionalism and quality. Their strategy in negotiations, however, reflected the continuing marginality of nursing issues within the health service, as they tended to speak rarely but to have been involved far more than medics in the drafting of the 'contract', and production of the written document.

Nursing concerns to some extent overlapped with those expressed by doctors, focusing largely on such issues as the information presented by management – that is, the managerial description of the service – and its validity. They sometimes took the opportunity presented by 'contract' negotiation to draw attention to problems connected with their part of the service and in some cases refused to sign the 'contract' unless these had been resolved. Discussions centred almost entirely on the number of interventions to be made during the following year as the figures held by clinical teams and those produced by managers differed. Whose information was right? And whose would be used? In addition, there was no clarity over how an intervention was to be either defined or measured. Attention might also be drawn to what clinicians perceived to be poor organisation: for example, the extended stays in hospital of generally elderly patients whose acute medical needs have been met but who remain occupying urgently needed beds as alternative provision for their continuing care is unavailable elsewhere in the health or social services.

Medical strategies in relation to the 'contract' and by implication the reform in general differed. Some saw the 'contract' process as an opening to raise problems, others ignored the process and refused to participate. A minority of consultants in high-tech expensive specialties adopted the language of managerialism, converting their specialties willingly into clinical directorates in the hope of gaining extra resources at the expense of other competing specialties elsewhere in the country. However, even in this case, it is unclear whether the consultants concerned had so much changed their underlying attitude as simply sought to become entrepreneurs within a changing system. Broadly, doctors in local services where there was no possibility of competition bringing in extra resources were least likely to show enthusiasm for the changes. However, where they did participate they tended to operate as mavericks. It was clear that, even where the clinical team had discussed the position they would hold during negotiations in relation to purchasers, medics were quite likely to express personal views which differed. This had the unintended effect of neatly throwing out managerial strategies for negotiations.

The managers, as we have seen, had strong agendas for the 'contract' process and the reform in general. However, unit management and clinical teams often had a long history of disagreement and suspicion behind them. Unit management, despite its new face, was unable to seize the initiative and act as advocate for clinical teams or the unit as a whole. For all managers, whether providers or purchasers, significant problems lay in the fact that only a tiny minority had any clinical training. They were constantly confronted with situations which they could not fully deal with and in addition were aware of the weakness of their own data. The purchasers' carefully co-ordinated strategies for negotiations were often thrown apart by medics who would not stick to the written agenda. As we shall see below, beyond these differences were interesting collusions of interest which were covert and unexpressed.

For purchasers, the 'contract' was a 'service agreement', that is, a description of the service, open to some degree of change during the year as situations altered. It was not necessary that it be signed by unit management or clinicians as it had no binding force. Yet in some way, everyone – clinical and managerial – clearly perceived that contracts did have some kind of significance, and gave the opportunity for gaining some leverage over situation or that they could be used to gain leverage. The ambiguities lie in the fact that neither workload figures incorporated into the document nor price reflect the health need or demand existing in the population and that the 'contract' does not in fact effect or shape that need or demand.

What is significant here is that what government and management in its official declarations envisage as a neutral process, an agreement over workload, quality and price, reflecting practice in the private sector – 'base-line service agreements that just described what was going on' (director of purchasing) – became in the health service a conflict over description, shaped by competing interests. Moreover, where there might be areas of agreement between managers and clinicians, the market model did not help to resolve problems, but became an inflexible one imposed on a reality which needed *more* communication between contrasting groups of professionals and institutions rather than less.

At a straightforward level within a single hospital, where resources had flowed between specialities as required – for example, the flexible use of beds – the 'contract' created a new rigidity where everything had to be codified and resources jealously guarded. In a more complex example, the market model was unable to resolve difficulties generated by existing boundaries between professional groups which each controlled resources. Where it was necessary for best practice in relation to service-users and for efficiency that resources be used flexibly across professional boundaries and domains, the use of 'contracts' proved cumbersome and incapable of dissolving boundaries. The 'contract' emphasises separation of resources and control rather than a more informal pooling of information, control and resources. This occurs in situations already characterised by the tendency to hold on to them in a situation of scarcity. Thus, for example, it proved impossible to resolve the situation described above of patients with needs for long-term care unnecessarily occupying high-tech beds in acute medicine. Access to community beds, the next step down in treatment, in some cases is controlled by GPs, and to some extent by nursing staff, who use them according to their own criteria and are unwilling to yield control over admission to the hospital service.

Dilemmas over patients and resources

For management, it was possible to talk about interventions which were appropriate and those which were not, and to include or exclude them from the range of treatments available to patients. Implicit in this view was the idea that need, far from being a passively existing condition in nature, is rather shaped and defined by clinicians. This view infuriated clinicians who saw 'disease' as a natural condition with its own pressing demands which can be postponed for a while, but ultimately must be met:

> As far as we're concerned the patients turn up at the front door to be treated and we cannot – I use the word front door both literally and conceptually – we cannot envisage a situation where we would say – sorry, your health District has only contracted for 30 people like you in a year and you're the 31st – tough. So we don't see health care delivery in those sort of terms. It's not us who generate the work, it's the disease and the patients who turn up. (Consultant)

> If there were not enough money there was some discussion about . . . the providers would have to advise the purchasers on which patients may be inappropriate to treat and our whole argument was that there

wouldn't be any patients that were inappropriate to treat when it came down to it . . . I mean, what do you do with these people who have a cancer diagnosis . . . ? Just sort of send them out on the streets and say, sorry we haven't got any money? But that was our concern. (Senior Nurse)

By the autumn and winter in many specialties the workload figures in the 'contracts' were shown to be inaccurate – the money had been spent, but the patients were still coming in. How was it to be decided who would receive health care? The discussions that took place then and the ways in which the difficulties were resolved indicate clearly the existence of conflicting definitions of the problem and corresponding uncertainty over responsibility for it and the appropriate response. Thus one consultant said: 'some people called it an overspend, we called it underfunding . . . Whose responsibility . . . that isn't entirely clear.' The problems were not new, but the new system is designed to eliminate the traditional response. In the past patients have been put on waiting lists based on the diagnostic decisions of clinicians, or doctors and nurses have decided which patients will be treated and in what ways using a combination of medical and social diagnoses and with a greater or lesser degree of involvement of the patient and family. The decisions over individual patients were never explicitly tied to resources.

Under the new system it is anticipated that clinical teams operating as service delivery units holding their own budgets and making contracts with people who want to buy health care – District purchasers, GPs, private patients – will decide what kinds of treatment they will offer within the resources available. In turn, purchasers will find out what health care their local population needs and buy it appropriately. Managers believe in a watered-down or explicit form of utilitarianism – the greatest good of the greatest number. In some London hospitals 'Quality Assessed Life Years' are used to determine who will get treatment, given scarce resources. Yet in practice this rational system remained unworkable – how can patients be turned away? Who will take the decision? It is both ethically and politically problematic.

In one emergency specialty, clinicians agreed that they could save money by not providing recently developed but expensive drugs which relieve illness without curing it, or by not treating certain categories of terminally ill patients, but they refused to take responsibility. They insisted that 'it would be a political decision' that the District Health Authority would have to announce publicly. Managers and clinical team agreed on a definition of the problem – underfunding, the responsibility for which lay with the government. It seemed an irresolvable situation and the senior nurse present suggested that together they present the case to the media. At this point the medics, who hitherto had been in apparently hostile confrontation with management, and management came together in turning down this proposal.

It is perhaps significant that it was a nurse, a member of a relatively marginal and largely female professional group within the health service hierarchy, who suggested breaking the pattern, opening up dilemmas to public awareness and challenging the political rules which play such a concealed and dominant part within what happens and is decided in health care. Instead, the dilemmas were resolved by a series of compromises such as the finding of small sums of money to tide over the situation and the managing of admissions. Market discipline did not come into play. As one consultant says: 'The system just about coped under very great pressure . . . it was coped with by incurring an overspend on nurse overtime and the nurse bank budget. And that is how . . . the health service struggles by in much of the country much of the time.' But more fundamentally, the dilemmas were not resolved explicitly in terms of a set of principles. Underneath the market language remains a commitment to providing health care to the individual patient and reliance on the authority of clinicians.

Needs assessment

In Year 1, purchasers had begun trying to implement the second and crucial role they had been given: they were to buy services on the basis of the health needs of their local population which they were to measure or assess. A complex series of meetings was set up involving professionals, consumer groups and service-users to consult on various areas where a shift in resources might improve the service, and a series of recommendations was drawn up. However, these areas, which were all ones where prevention might reduce costs in the acute sector, were of no immediate pressing concern compared to the problems in certain acute specialties. At the end of the year it was decided by purchasers that any extra money should go into acute care and the needs assessment fell by the wayside. To quote the Director of Purchasing commenting on the fact that they value health promotion and community services: 'when you look at the way we spend our money, it doesn't actually match the values'.

But needs assessment is problematic for other reasons. The legislation is built on assumptions about need, information, technical know-how and competition. In this view, need exists out there in the population and simply has to be assessed through the use of scientific methods. But need is rather an interaction between various factors including the knowledge of the population about treatment which could be available, the effectiveness of intervention, the fairness of intervention. How to determine whose needs are to be met and on what criteria – those of individuals or of particular groups of individuals, such as the elderly, or children; those suffering from particular conditions; or particular communities, such as the most disadvantaged?

Who should collect the information – the legislation envisaged a Public Health Department providing information to purchasers, but this foundered on the micro-politics of the relation between the Public Health doctors and purchaser. Purchasers envisaged Public Health as playing an advisory role as and when they required information, but the doctors themselves argued that they were not the 'handmaidens' of the purchasers but an autonomous centre of expertise. Consultants argued that their own waiting-lists were an indicator of need. Then community clinicians stressed the wishes the population had actually made in open meetings – which were for more hip replacements and chiropody, neither of which were high on the priority list of the purchasers (in the latter case, at the bottom).

Information then in reality is shown not to be a neutral resource, but one which is used, and which became an instrument within a struggle for resources and between systems of knowledge and power. Managers felt a 'power imbalance' working with clinical teams and were afraid that perhaps they got a biased view. Yet purchasers did not know how they could obtain a fair picture of the dilemmas they faced over resource allocation. *Ad hoc* advisory groups tended to multiply as each interest group demanded representation, to the point that they were unable to achieve consensus. Small groups in the new style of management, composed only of those considered the most able to find a decision, were considered unrepresentative by those excluded. To consult members of the specialty concerned, purchasers felt, would result in bias, but would it be appropriate 'to go to a radiotherapist for a view on mental health'? (Director of Purchasing). Under these circumstances they placed great emphasis on language, often ironically contrasting the tasks laid on them by 'on high' with the realities of managing the health

service on a day-to-day basis. Thus in one discussion between purchasers the statement 'equal access as a principle of purchasing' was
revised to 'access to health care for all patients according to health
care need'; the term 'comprehensive' was questioned because 'it's
never going to be entirely comprehensive because we have got to
make choices' and the word 'appropriate' was suggested ironically
instead.

Conclusion

The problems which arose between managers and clinical teams
derived in part from a failure to communicate and the effects of
using different languages. There sometimes seemed to be areas of
agreement and opportunities for action and change which were not
taken, because neither side could understand or accept the language
used by the other. If managers were more ready to use a language of
individual patient-centred care, they might find more acceptance
from clinicians. The gulf which clinicians often felt existed between
themselves and management was reinforced by what they saw as the
reluctance of many managers to go on to the wards and see the
realities of sickness and death and the problems which, they believe,
are caused by lack of resources. Clinicians felt that managers isolated
themselves from the reality of the decisions they took over resources, passing on the responsibility for rationing health care to doctors
and nurses. Some clinicians felt that to expect doctors and nurses to
take the cost of treatment into consideration when deciding whether
an intervention was appropriate for a given patient would erode the
relationship of trust between clinician and patient. Yet here there
was a failure on the part of purchasing managers to establish clearly
their own boundaries of responsibility, which included the setting of
priorities and decisions over what health care to buy.

The fundamental question is whether managers possess special
knowledge which both they and clinicians feel to be valid and
worthy of respect in the same way as medical knowledge. Secondly,
there is a need for managers to show clinicians that they do understand the outlook of doctors and nurses, which is rooted in the
immediate relationship with the individual patient and the details of
daily life on the ward or in the clinic or practice. Purchasing managers, in particular, face highly complex situations in which different
professional and lay interest groups compete to maintain control
over resources or to shape the way in which health care is provided.

Until purchasers establish clear policies, their failure to resolve problems (such as that described previously of continuing care for the elderly infirm) even after long-drawn-out processes of consultation, deprives purchaser management of any authority in the eyes both of clinicians and of unit managers.

At present, the situation is unclear, with purchasing management unsure over its policy, and its decisions producing unexpected and unintended consequences on other aspects of the service. Financial imperatives reflected in the setting of 'contracts' and the choices made by GP fund holders begin to affect specialties, compelling some to contract, others to expand. Unit managers, particularly trust managers, on the other hand, feel that they possess a new authority in relation both to purchasers and to clinical teams as those responsible for the organisation and financial well-being of 'the corporate hospital' or unit. Clinicians, on the other hand, may feel increasingly frustrated and prone to withdraw from any involvement in the organisational side of the health service, as their perceptions are ignored.

What then are the implications and consequences for the service-user? In theory the reform offers a new brand of paternalism in which an elite of managers and clinicians who have adopted the managerial role decide who will receive health care. In practice, we have seen a great deal of confusion over what kind of health care should be provided, and a great deal of rhetoric. In prticular, the responsibility for rationing health care or, in other words, establishing priorities, has not been clarified. The perceptions and needs of the service-user are very different from those that preoccupy managers and clinicians. Although one strand of the reform is concerned with collecting the views of the user and the public in general, it is essential that this voice is added to the debate in a much stronger form.

There is no perfect answer in regard to the provision of health care, and the dilemmas are complex and difficult. Ultimately, we shall benefit from greater clarity in regard to the decisions made in the health service, and from a wider understanding of the issues that affect medicine and care. It is necessary to go beyond narrow professional interests and identities to focus on how aspects of care interact, and to discuss the best ways in which care can be provided. Such an approach starts from the patient-centred model of health care and avoids the ethically unacceptable and politically unworkable promises of utilitarianism whilst opening up exploration of how the individual patient is situated within a potential network of care.

References

Burke K. (1969), *A Rhetoric of Motives* (Berkeley: University of California Press).

Foucault, M. (1963), *The Birth of the Clinic* (London: Tavistock).

Geertz, C. (1973), *The Interpretation of Cultures* (London: Hutchinson).

Gramsci, A. (1971), *Selections from Prison Notebooks* (London: Lawrence & Wishart).

Harden, I. (1992), *The Contracting State* (Buckingham: Open University Press).

Harrison, S., Hunter, D.J. and Pollitt, C. (1990), *The Dynamics of British Health Policy* (London: Unwin Hyman).

Hughes, D. (1991), 'The reorganisation of the National Health Service: The rhetoric and reality of the internal market', *Modern Law Review*, 54, pp. 88–103.

Klein, R. (1983), *The Politics of the NHS* (London: Longman).

Lakoff G. and Johnson, M. (1980), *Metaphors We Live By* (Chicago: University of Chicago Press).

Strong, P. and Robinson, J. (1990), *The NHS – Under New Management* (Buckingham: Open University Press).

Weber, M. (1976), *The Protestant Ethic and the Spirit of Capitalism* (London: Allen & Unwin).

Interprofessional collaboration in action

5 *Elderly care*

Gail Wilson and Julie Dockrell

Chapter summary

The authors focus on the complexity of professional advice and support associated with services for elderly people; they continue the theme of the earlier chapters of dissolving public service systems which are outside professional control. The introduction of multidisciplinary assessments and packages of care is discussed in the context of interprofessional collaboration. The authors draw upon their research material on professional perceptions of their own and others' work and practice. They examine the importance of interprofessional collaboration, and the negative and potentially destructive effects of competition and a market philosophy in health and social care for this client group.

Introduction

Recent government legislation has had a dramatic effect on the organisation and planning of services for older people. The move to make the social services department the lead authority in co-ordinating community care for frail older people has altered the locus of responsibility for service provision. Moreover, the split between purchasers and providers of care involves major changes in the delivery and funding of services. The structure of existing services is changing. At the same time, the government intends the independent sector – both private and voluntary – to take a much greater part in providing basic services. Under the new legislation individual service-users will have a professionally designed care package, and professionals will monitor and reassess care delivery. The local social services department, as the enabling authority, will set up inspection units to monitor standards in the private and voluntary care sectors as well as social services. Community and hospital-based services remain outside these monitoring arrangements, but are expected to co-operate in providing care and in multidisciplinary assessments.

Different types of professional have for historical reasons become concentrated in different services. Training has mirrored service divisions, but many of the skills needed to care for frail elderly people are common to a wide range of professionals and non-professionals. If services based on the needs of individuals become a reality, it will be increasingly hard to justify existing professional divisions. The intended growth of the private and voluntary sectors will also threaten traditional professional divides. More trained staff will be needed by private care organisations and voluntary agencies as they compete for local authority care contracts, or sell their services to GP fundholders and other health service purchasers. However, these professionals will be recruited as care providers rather than as members of health or social services.

The new activity is both stimulating and a challenge to professionals in the caring services, but the changes take place against a background which is outside professional control. First there is the demographic imperative. The number of people over 80 is due to rise by 50 per cent over the next decade. Changes in family and labour force mean that female relatives may not be present or willing to offer the increasing number of frail older people as much support as they have done in the past. If the family cannot provide adequate support, formal care services must make up the short-fall. Caring for older people in the community is not a cheap option and more frail elders will mean higher expenditure. However, the National Health Service and Community Care Act was designed to reduce per capita expenditure on frail elders, not increase it. The inescapable logic is that, without extra money, services will be increasingly stretched in the future. Estes and Swan (1993) have already identified a 'care gap' in the USA. We can expect similar developments in the UK.

The ideal needs-led service for the varied group of people who make up the user group known as 'the elderly,' would allow for individual specification in line with individual needs. This is in essence the aim of the new policies. The new services will be able to take account of complex and changing conditions in the life of older people. Such an aim implies a service that is not delivered in standardised units, but can be tailor-made for each user and/or carer – a comprehensive assessment followed by the planned delivery of individual packages of care. Given the range of needs among users, such a service has to be multidisciplinary, but the number of disciplines and the types of organisation involved can vary widely.

While in theory the new developments could provide greater choice, in practice the changes highlight a range of interorganisational problems which may restrict choice. If the changes result in more rigid boundaries between professionals, it is possible for gaps in service provision to grow. Once service responsibilities are clearly defined some people will always fall outside the limits. Older people are particularly vulnerable because their needs cross professional and organisational boundaries. The success or failure of multidisciplinary and inter-agency working has specific repercussions on the care that is provided for them.

This chapter begins with an analysis of the stereotypes and barriers to joint working. We then highlight the multiple needs of older people and move on to consider the ways in which multiple needs interact with professional paradigms and organisational issues. The term 'professional paradigms' is here intended to signify the attitudes and values which groups of professionals hold about themselves and about other professions. We conclude by considering ways of overcoming some of the problems which have been identified.

There is a danger that analyses of interprofessional working by outsiders will suggest values and orientations that do not exist in working practice. In so doing, they may create unhelpful stereotypes. We therefore began our analysis by turning to the workers themselves and asking how professional paradigms impinged on their working practices. Over the last two years we have asked groups of practitioners from various backgrounds to identify the ways in which their daily work practices were affected by both explicit and implicit professional assumptions. The comments generated from these discussions inform our analysis.

Professional paradigms

Community care attempts to offer frail older people the opportunity of living as independent a life as possible within cost constraints. Services need to involve many professionals and to cross professional boundaries. Community services fall into six main categories: relatives and friends (informal carers); local authority social services; local health services; independent (private and voluntary) sector services; local housing department services; and transport. Local health services will include a range of professionals such as district nurses, health visitors, occupational therapists, clinical psychologists, community psychiatric nurses and general practitioners. Each professional will provide a different approach from a different training base.

From the point of view of the user it is often unclear which of these many professionals is providing a service. This confusion is perhaps inevitable as long as the boundaries between professions are based on a mixture of historical accident and professional practice rather than tasks performed (Normand, 1993). Not surprisingly, service-users are often confused or unaware about what is on offer (Allen *et al.*, 1992). As one of the clients in this study said, 'You hear of things. It's like this – people gossip. You have to keep your wits about you. I'm quick on the uptake . . .' (p. 80). The users surveyed generally felt that they were not well informed. They failed to receive information about the services available and specific information about their own health status, particularly from general practitioners.

For the professionals, the implications of a multi-provider environment and interprofessional working are often more subtle. At one level it is clear that health services should respond to the 'health' needs of the individual and social services to the 'social' needs. In later life it can become very difficult to define these differences clearly and with so many providers, it is often difficult to work out who should do what and who should pay for what. Disputes about responsibility are likely to increase.

How can effective working be supported? The first step to such understanding is to identify explicitly the professional differences that exist. It will then become possible to address the issues of difference and to ameliorate their impact on services for users.

As a start we asked small groups of practitioners from similar backgrounds to identify the assumptions they felt characterised their professional activities. We worked with professionals with backgrounds in nursing, social work, social care and a range of other disciplines. Some groups of professionals were underrepresented (for example, housing managers) and some were entirely absent (for example, occupational therapists and general practitioners). The groups were composed of professionals who had chosen to attend management of community care courses and hence were not specially chosen for the purpose of the study. The participants came from three different service sectors: the health services, social services and the voluntary sector.

Each of our groups represented workers who had continuing direct contact with older people, either in designing or delivering services. Nurses of different specialities and grades were mainly from the health service. Social services were represented by trained social workers and residential and other care staff. The voluntary and private sectors included nurses and others who originated from a range of different backgrounds. Some of them identified professionally with the health or social service staff, but the majority identified themselves by sector rather than profession.

Single discipline groups first identified professional stereotypes, their own and their views of others. These stereotypes were then fed back to all participants. At the second stage the groups were reconstituted into mixed professional/sector groups and considered ways of addressing potential conflicts.

Our three groups identified seven potential areas of difference: language used; organisation of services and the professional hierarchy; the definition of the service-users; needs of the service-users; class; ethnicity; and ideology. To a large extent, the differences identified in stage one reflected the ideology inherent in the different training processes. These opinions inform our opening analysis.

Participants coming from a health background tended to locate their professional frameworks or stereotypes within a range of nursing models. Specifically they talked about the importance of the nurses' uniform as an indication of their status and the need to keep patient notes confidential. They explicitly called their service-users *patients*. There was a great deal of emphasis on the formality of a service, providing care and treatment to *patients* and basing professional decisions on the knowledge of correct procedures. They highlighted the importance of the nurses' training in qualifying them to identify patients' needs. In particular, they emphasised older people's need for accurate diagnoses, an area in which they were qualified as a result of their training. They tended to explain failures of the prescribed interventions in terms of patient non-compliance. Despite the fact that the majority of our respondents were now working in the community their professional framework tended to be hospital-based.

In contrast, those from the social services placed great emphasis on designing services *for groups of clients*, seeing themselves as the gatekeepers to a range of services, such as meals on wheels or day care, which they allocated as appropriate. They viewed service failures in terms of restrictions on resources. They saw themselves as in tune with the needs of the community, in contrast to health services staff, whom they perceived as being out of touch with community needs. Their professional status was enhanced by running or guiding a team. The social services staff also placed less emphasis on the individual than did staff from the health sector. It was clear that much of their professional autonomy had been reduced by legislative demands on social services generally. Thus, for generic social workers, the impact of the Children Act 1989 influenced the way their time was allocated and their access to resources. The statutory requirements of other service areas produced specific organisational constraints which restricted the resources allocated to older people.

The voluntary sector was, to a large extent, excluded from these professional arrangements. Staff saw themselves as marginalised both by their lack of formal training and the limited control they exercised over resources. They felt like the poor sister to the other powerful agencies. Despite this perception, morale was high. They saw training as a critical element in achieving professional status. Some of the voluntary workers were trained professionals, but on the whole they came from outside the disciplines related to human services. There was an implicit assumption in the group that the term 'professional' could only be equated with possession of a recognised qualification. By this definition staff in non-statutory agencies were often not professionals. While the voluntary sector staff saw their role as empowering service-users, they regarded themselves as peripheral to decision-making with respect to the allocation of funds and the development of services. They felt that they were continually fighting for resources and that these exchanges took place outside any formal structures.

The group discussions and presentations back to all the participants showed that interprofessional issues can be both overt and covert. It was clear that the explicit level of analysis masked a range of implicit issues which impinged on the way that different professionals saw themselves, their futures and their professional practices. There was a tacit acknowledgement that promotion needed to occur through the professional hierarchy. This entailed possessing and using a particular set of professional skills in a particular domain. Being the expert did not lend itself to sharing skills or relinquishing responsibility to other workers in a different sector.

Needs-led multidisciplinary services require shared skills and a move away from traditional organisationally-based professional divisions. Skills become the critical factor, not professional training. Thus, staff in both health and social services realised that their power of decision-making was under threat and that their future professional roles were unclear. They might view the voluntary and private sectors as 'amateur' or even with contempt, because many of these services employ untrained staff and, in the private sector, are out for financial gain. On the other hand, there was also a fear that a better service, addressing clients' needs, might be on offer.

There is a danger that staff who feel threatened will withdraw behind professional barriers. They may also stress other aspects of status such as class, race and gender. A key finding from our interprofessional groups was the need to consider whether status differences between qualified and unqualified staff were valid in elder care. The recognition of the skills and strengths which all well-motivated staff can offer to users is a first step to mutual respect. However, goodwill cannot be assumed when so many staff feel threatened. Areas of conflict and potential conflict need to be identified and solutions negotiated.

The range of needs of older people

Older people who become users of health or social care services tend to have accumulated a wide range of needs before they are referred to service agencies. A responsive service should take a comprehensive approach to the assessment of need and this is the aim of the new legislation. There is still a risk that professionals will see needs in terms of their initial training and so take a narrow view of user strengths and weaknesses. Other pressures will reinforce such a trend. In the future, as numbers rise of people in the age groups when they are most likely to become frail (over 80), and finance fails to increase at the same rate (one purpose of the NHS and Community Care Act), there will be growing pressure on resources. Providers will find it necessary to prioritise their services in terms of risk rather than quality of life or user satisfaction. However, risks are usually defined in terms of services needed or the professional training needed to identify them. For example, there can be medical risks, psychological risks, social risks and economic risks. It may well become difficult to maintain a comprehensive approach if funding becomes a battle between particular risks or risk groups.

A high quality service can only be provided if all professionals recognise that the needs of men and women in later life are complex. Practice needs to take account of this complexity. The necessary knowledge and skills range from a basic core, which should be common to all professionals, to the highly specialised (for example, monitoring drug intakes).

All staff need to be able to combat ageist stereotypes and to understand that frail elders have long life-histories and varied needs. People in later life are the victims of prejudices and ageist beliefs that frequently combine to make them feel devalued as human beings and a burden on society (Victor, 1987). While most older people are able to overcome these prejudices in their daily lives, they often feel devalued when they come into contact with caring professionals. For example, in one survey the main complaint of service-users was that they were not treated with respect (Wilson, 1993).

It follows that one of the greatest needs of all older service-users is to be treated with respect and as worthwhile individuals. All contacts between users and professionals should ideally be marked by mutual respect, but more effort is needed for older people who are so persistently devalued by ageist beliefs in society. Ageism is a problem for professionals working with older people and their carers. Practitioners are not immune from ageist beliefs and need to examine their own unconscious biases against their client group. One way of maintaining high morale and a high quality service is for staff to see themselves as advocates for older people in the face of an ageist and often uncaring society.

People in later life are usually referred to by collective nouns, 'elderly', 'older people', 'elders', 'the old' (as in this chapter). There may be little attempt to differentiate needs on the basis of age, gender or ethnicity. Old age does not begin at retirement but many services take 60 or 65 as the cut-off point for their client group. It is not uncommon for women to live for thirty years after retiring from paid work – the same lifespan as from fifteen to forty-five. No one would class fifteen year-olds with forty-five year-olds, but older people are routinely lumped together regardless of age. Familial caregivers are typically either spouses or children. Both may be past retirement age, but professionals will find that the needs of caregivers who are daughters or sons in their sixties will be very different from spouses in their eighties.

Services for the elderly often imply that gender differences are no longer important. Commonly held gender stereotypes no longer apply in old age. Older men are rarely full-time workers and older women are not mothers, though many of the younger generation of elders help with childcare. Men may become carers (Arber and Gilbert, 1989) and women may find themselves managing the finances or changing fuses. The needs of men and women will still differ, but not necessarily in the ways currently recognised by professionals. Women, with their higher levels of chronic illness (Victor, 1991) and greater mobility problems, could benefit from more help than they receive. Men, on the other hand, might be encouraged to be more adaptable and to help themselves.

Ethnic differences are a serious challenge to our caring services in the 1990s. Ethnic minorities who arrived in different periods and for different reasons are rapidly approaching ages where the chances of disability increase. They are reaching old age without the traditional support they might have expected. Family networks have been very much reduced by migration in some cases. In others, relatives find it hard to care because they are themselves suffering from the very low incomes, reduced pensions, poor health and poor housing that accompany racial discrimination.

Ethnic minority elders may find it hard to use the caring services. Language problems may reduce the amount of information they have. A history of migration and racial discrimination can present special mental health problems in old age. Even more important, the services themselves are often of little use to ethnic minority elders (Bowling, 1990). They rarely take account of the specific needs of different groups, for example, for special diets or religious observation. Many ethnic elders belong to cultures where the roles of men and women are more clearly differentiated than among native elders. They may need separate provision for men and women. Most will need separate provision away from the racism of majority elders whenever it is possible. Professionals from different backgrounds urgently need to pool their knowledge at both organisational and individual level if they are to respond appropriately to ethnic elders. The range of linguistic, religious and cultural needs of older men and women from ethnic minorities far exceeds the existing knowledge base of service providers.

Although many professionals from a medical or nursing background will be well aware that much can be done to remedy ill health in advanced old age, others may need reminding that old age does not equal physical or mental frailty. Professionals are hardly to blame for having a limited view of health in old age. They rarely see normal active elders and their elder friends and relatives may be the only healthy members of the age group that they meet. However, health is a vital aspect of well-being and quality of life in old age. All professionals working with older people need as much knowledge of preventive health care and common conditions as possible so that they can refer users on to proper medical care. General practitioners, in particular, may find it hard to accept that they do not know enough about geriatric medicine to serve the full range of their patients.

Housing is frequently unmentioned in professional training courses. This is an important omission, because home is where the majority of older people spend a very great deal of their time. Home conditions can be disabling or enabling. A good service will not leave housing problems to the occupational therapist. All professionals will be aware of basic problems like steps, badly designed switches and shelves. There are other aspects of housing more closely related to self-esteem and quality of life. Men or women who can no longer decorate their homes or keep their gardens respectable may feel degraded and lack motivation.

Any problems with housing will be intensified by low income. Money can buy so many necessities in old age and make up for so many limitations. It is not uncommon to find that rising rents and council tax demands leave frail elderly people with little money for food or heating. Health problems are more or less inevitable in such circumstances but many professionals are not trained to consider financial circumstances. A basic training in benefits rights and good relations with the local Citizen's Advice Bureau are part of the essential base for all who work with older people.

Many older people were not able to get much education when they were young. This does not mean they cannot learn, but it may mean that they are easily impressed by educational qualifications in others. Overstressed professionals may sometimes be glad of deferential users, but the new community care is based on the premise of partnership. The aim is for users to develop their abilities for self-care. For example, there is a common assumption that widowers need high levels of service because they do not know how to cook and clean. The only alternative offered may be a move to residential care. In fact there is no evidence that older people cannot learn new skills as long as they see the point of the exercise (Bromley, 1990). Widowers can learn to cook, but if they are given services on a permanent basis rather than as a rehabilitative measure, they have little chance to show what they can do.

The National Health Service and Community Care Act 1990 marks a shift in government policy in favour of informal caregivers. The aim is to help caregivers to continue and so economise on scarce services. Professionals therefore have to take into account the diverse needs of caregivers in a more systematic way than before. Different professionals view caregivers in different ways. General practitioners, for example, were trained to consider the patient as an individual (Atkin and Twigg, 1991). Social work on the other hand has stressed the family as a unit: social workers have tended towards a family model when working with older people. It has been argued that those working in the voluntary sector often consider the wider needs of the community. Interprofessional services have to take account of these differences in professional perceptions of users and compensate for them in ways that do not affect the quality of services delivered.

Local conditions are also important. Long distances between centres, thinly spread services and poor public transport make for special problems in rural areas. Unsafe housing estates, traffic congestion and poor living conditions result in special problems in some highly stressed urban areas. At present frail elders are concentrated in declining inner city areas and retirement towns. In the inner cities deprivation is the norm and younger relatives who had the chance have migrated to better areas. In retirement towns relatives may have been left behind and the sheer number of pensioners is a strain on health and social services. In future, the main concentrations of older people are likely to be on the fringes of towns, in the housing estates and suburbs that were built before and after the Second World War. Services are easier to provide when users are close together. Scattered elders, and in particular scattered members of ethnic minority groups, make service provision expensive.

The impact of professional boundaries on service provision

Organisational complexity is a fact of life for staff. The challenge is to reduce its adverse impact on users. From the point of view of the elderly service user or her relatives, many services mean many points of entry. The professional label on the service door has a great effect on the service received (Hunter *et al.*, 1988). It is quite possible for a carer looking after a mentally frail husband or wife to find that the community psychiatric nurse will offer support in terms of counselling, mental health education and relaxation techniques. The same couple might find that social services recognised the need for a break by the offer of a day centre place. If they were very lucky, they might get a sitting service when referred to the voluntary sector. They may have been assessed for each service, but the perception of need and the remedies offered are the product of professional training, as well as service organisation and availability.

In theory, multidisciplinary assessment will overcome these difficulties. In practice, assessment is only a first step. The design and monitoring of individual packages of care mean that knowledge of all the services available – health and social, public, private and voluntary – has to be shared. The statutory services in our study had little awareness of the organisation and accountability of their non-statutory colleagues. Flexibility and choice will only begin to be a reality for users when one professional is as likely as any other to recommend a place in a day hospital or a private domiciliary carer.

The multidisciplinary groups reported on above felt that communication was the key to successful interdisciplinary working. Liaison and joint planning are essential and language is the medium for these activities. There was general agreement that professional jargon can hamper communication and should be reduced. In spite of this agreement, individuals recognised that the elimination of professional terminology might reduce their professional status. How do professionals retain their identity if everyone uses the same words? Once again, fears for status endanger interprofessional co-operation.

However, using the same words is not a panacea. As our multidisciplinary groups clearly illustrated, different professions meant different things, even though they used the same words. The term 'service-user' is a case in point. The term may refer to the index patient, the family, other service agencies or the community in general. 'Community' may be thought of primarily as 'the place where clients live' or as 'a workplace which is not a hospital'. One suggestion for avoiding communication difficulties was to develop trust between the professionals concerned. It was not clear how trust could be developed in a competitive market.

The new emphasis on managed markets (Le Grand, 1991), will increase the possibility of competition between service organisations and make co-operative working even more difficult. Suggestions made by our groups such as the pooling of resources, will not be possible in a market situation. Joint planning, another suggested solution, has been in effect since the 1970s and has not solved the problem of co-ordination. The new emphasis on joint assessment could improve interprofessional communication but is potentially very time-consuming. A further problem is that the criteria for joint assessment have to be negotiated so that the assessment forms are owned by all the professionals concerned or they will not be properly used.

In the future, users who need high cost services or who are very difficult to deal with, may find their needs are not met. In a market environment services will have to make a profit or keep within a given contract price. Professionals may find themselves under pressure to drop expensive users or to refer them to another agency. If competition between agencies increases, there will also be a growth in secrecy and suspicion between staff in different services. It will become more difficult for professionals to exchange vital information about users.

Even if an increase in the more destructive aspects of marketisation can be avoided, it is certain that in the future services will have to be targeted towards those in greatest need (Davies *et al.*, 1990). However, targeting involves defining service boundaries more clearly and setting strict eligibility criteria. More people have to be defined as ineligible, even though they have service needs.

Traditionally, the role of the voluntary sector has been to fill such gaps in formal health and social services. This will be more difficult in the future, because the voluntary sector is likely to be fully stretched doing some of the work which was once done by statutory agencies. Moreover, voluntary sector organisations themselves may have clear ideas of their role in service provision. They may decide not to compensate for the gaps left by statutory services.

Gaps in service delivery have been theorised in two ways. In the first, the boundaries of different agencies harden and it becomes more difficult to work outside them. Professionals may or may not work co-operatively within their organisations but market competition makes them unwilling to work with others in outside agencies. Two problems arise: in some cases potential service-users with multiple needs will fail to get the types and amounts of service they need; in others there will be duplication of services with a consequent waste of resources. Professionals from different agencies will find it hard to work together.

The second and more positive approach to the problem of gaps sees the space between services acting as a vacuum and sucking in the commitment of concerned professionals. According to this model, services stay separate but they have enough flexibility to allow their staff to work across boundaries and to liaise and co-operate with similarly motivated staff from other agencies. Real interprofessional work thus results. The problem with this model is that it relies on special conjunctions of concerned professionals. They must have the personal skills, knowledge and motivation to work outside the official boundaries of their agencies with other professionals who are similarly motivated. These conditions will not be met everywhere. We cannot therefore assume that interprofessional work will automatically follow from present developments.

Conclusion

Older people themselves are not a homogeneous group. They differ according to age, gender, ethnic group, and health status. Any health and social care needs they have are often complicated by poor housing, low income and limited education. Their informal carers may similarly vary, with a major distinction in needs between younger generation carers, who are mainly female, and same generation carers who may be husbands or wives.

It follows that the health and social care needs of older people are varied and complex. Practitioners who provide services to older people have skills that have been historically defined by different training and professional pathways. Often they work in separate health and social care agencies or in the voluntary or private sectors. Users frequently do not understand these divisions, but they may suffer from them.

Overlapping health and social care services imply professionals who can share their skills. However, this can only be done when morale is high and different professions do not feel threatened by others. Given that society places a low social value on older people and on those who look after them, professionals must be prepared to combat ageism in all aspects of their practice as a first step to improved morale.

The practitioners who took part in the study reported here saw barriers between professionals as related to differences in the use of language; in organisational structure; in ways of defining service-users; in understanding of users' needs; in service ideology and in class, gender and ethnicity. All these can lead to divisions between services which can result in gaps or duplication.

They identified better communications as a key to better services for elderly people. At one level, this involved changes in service structures to allow time for formal and informal contacts. At another level, it meant paying specific attention to the different meanings which different professions attach to common terms such as 'user' or 'community' and a conscious attempt to avoid professional jargon.

There was no single prescription for interprofessional working. Local solutions are essential because the environment where older people live has a direct impact on interprofessional work. However, there were some general principles. In the first place, it is well understood that professionals who co-operate will improve services for their users. This potential for improvement is enshrined in the National Health Service and Community Care Act 1990 which assumes that inter-agency and interprofessional work will take place. In the second, covert and often unrecognised forces that work against co-operation have to be explicitly recognised and dealt with. They include professional insecurities of all types ranging from concerns with promotion if cross-agency work is allowed, to feelings of being deskilled if jargon cannot be used. At an institutional level service boundaries have to be negotiated in ways that conform to budgets and minimise damage to users.

All staff, and not simply higher managers, need to recognise and work against the pressure to compete embodied in new developments of managed markets. Shortage of funds and the pressure to work competitively in a quasi-market place are likely to reinforce professional divisions unless conscious attempts to oppose them through joint training and similar events are made. Individual professionals will find it increasingly difficult to focus on the clients' needs when they are presented with a divergence of professional goals and organisational practices which restrict access to other disciplines.

The variations between individual older people can easily be overlooked when they are reduced to a category such as 'high dependency' or 'high risk'. However, it is essential to understand the effect of individual life histories and individual attributes in designing high quality, needs-led services. No one professional will have all the skills to recognise, let alone meet, the range and variety of needs presented by elderly service-users. It follows that interprofessional communication and shared service provision is not just a desirable addition in elderly care; it is an essential part of a quality service wherever that service is located and however it is organised.

References

Allen, I., Hogg, D. and Peace, S. (1992), *Elderly People: Choice participation and satisfaction* (London: Policy Studies Institute).

Arber, S. and Gilbert, N. (1989), 'Men: the forgotten carers', *Sociology*, 23, 1, pp. 111–18.

Atkin, K. and Twigg, J. (1991), 'General Practice and Informal Care: Assumptive worlds and embedded policies', Paper delivered at the British Society of Gerontology Conference, Manchester, 1991.

Bowling, B. (1990), *Elderly People from Ethnic Minorities: A Report on Four Projects* (London: Kings College Age Concern Institute of Gerontology).

Bromley, D.B. (1990), *Behavioural Gerontology: Central issues in the psychology of ageing* (Chichester: John Wiley).

Davies, B., Bebbington, A. and Charnley, H. (1990), *Resources, Needs and Outcomes* (Aldershot: Avebury).

Estes, C., and Swan, J.H. (1993), *The Long Term Care Crisis: Elders Trapped in the No Care Zone* (London: Sage).

Hunter, D. J., McKeganney, N. P. and MacPherson, I. (1988), *Care of the Elderly Policy and Practice* (Aberdeen: University of Aberdeen Press).

Le Grand, J. (1991), 'Quasi-markets and Social Policy', *Economic Journal*, 101, 408, pp. 1256–67.

Normand, C. E. M. (1993) 'Changing patterns of care: the challenge for health care professions and professionals', in M. Malek and P. Vaconi (eds), *Managerial Issues in Health Care Management* (Chicester: John Wiley and Co.).

Victor, C. (1987), *Old Age in Modern Society* (London: Croom Helm).

Victor C. (1991), *Health and Health Care in Later Life* (Milton Keynes: Open University Press).

Wilson G. (1993), 'Users and Providers: Different Perspectives on Community Care Services', *Journal of Social Policy*, vol. 22, no. 4.

6 *Child protection*

Elizabeth Birchall

Chapter summary

This chapter is based upon the author's original research and describes the different approaches of professional groups and agencies to the problem of child abuse. High standards of interprofessional co-ordination and collaboration in this area of social care is considered a priority by government, and the establishment of measures to promote such co-operation are outlined in detail. The roles, attitudes and constraints experienced by the different professionals involved are analysed and illustrated by the use of case studies.

Introduction

This chapter draws on a research project on 'Co-ordination in Child Protection' funded by the Department of Health and carried out by Christine Hallett and Elizabeth Birchall at the University of Stirling between 1988 and 1992 (Hallett and Birchall, 1992). Following an extensive literature review empirical work was undertaken in several diverse locations in the north of England. Methods used were a random sample survey, a case records study and interviews with the professionals involved in those cases. The detailed results have been presented in Birchall (1992) and Hallett (1993).

For many years the importance of interprofessional co-ordination has been a truism among eminent practitioners and policy-makers in the field of child protection. It has been a prominent feature of professional writings since Kempe *et al.* (1962) first caught professional attention in the United States with their seminal article on 'the battered child'. Particular emphasis has been placed on co-operation between social services, education, law enforcement, primary health and paediatric agencies. Psychiatric, psychological and other counselling agencies with a psychotherapeutic orientation have been less prominent in the official guidance on case management and in the practice network. The extent to which such agencies may recognise and manage problems which might be characterised as child abuse separately from the main network is obscure. There has been a marked emphasis on the identification and reporting of children who are victims or are at risk of abuse. However, there are other countries which have stressed the importance of client confidentiality and a voluntaristic approach to intervention as an encouragement to self-reporting and, therefore in their view, ultimately to more effective intervention (Christopherson, 1989).

The discussion in this chapter is focused upon mainstream practice in the UK, which has been particularly influenced by the American literature and more recently by British work such as Dale *et al.* (1986) and the Department of Health manual *Protecting Children: a guide for social workers undertaking a comprehensive assessment* (1988). Nevertheless, the fact that other countries have approached the issue from significantly different standpoints should not be forgotten.

Different approaches

Three perspectives from organisational sociology on interorganisational relations appear particularly relevant to the development of policy in the sphere of child protection. Two of these perspectives – exchange (Levine and White, 1961) and power/resource dependency (Aldrich, 1972, 1976, 1979; Benson, 1975) – evidently overlap, in that both show organisations forming lateral relationships for mutual benefit. Such benefits can include, for instance, the sharing of skills and reassurance as well as economy and efficiency in service delivery. However, a significant difference is that in the first case an equality of power may give both organisations equal control over the choice of costs and benefits while, in the second, a single organisation may determine the rewards to itself and the penalties of noncompliance to the subordinate partner.

The third perspective – mandated co-ordination (Hauf, 1978) – is more distinct, bringing in an external superior force which requires the collateral agencies to co-operate in situations where they may perceive insufficient shared interests or have insufficient differentials of power to establish effective relationships between themselves.

It is evident from the stream of increasingly detailed central government guidance, since the Tunbridge Wells Study Group (DHSS, 1973) and the concurrent Maria Colwell Inquiry (Colwell Report, 1974), continuing up to the latest edition of *Working Together* (Department of Health, 1991), that mandated co-ordination is a very prominent element in the British arena of child protection. Even so, the other perspectives have considerable bearing on everyday practice and, as Hallett and Birchall argue, on the development of that official guidance. While the guidance is 'founded upon the dominant understanding about the importance of an interagency response, essentially developed from voluntary exchanges between professionals and agencies' (1992, p. 38), the creation and maintenance of practical collaboration would also be affected by concepts such as domain consensus, power and status.

Moreover, they point out that organisations, local and central, do not exist in a social or political vacuum, nor do they exist separately from the people who work in them. Their structures and their goals are affected by a complex range of influences within the agencies and without. These are discussed in Section One of the present volume and, with particular reference to child protection, in Hallett and Birchall (1992). Five contrasting illustrations must suffice here: the independent contractor status jealously guarded by general practitioners; the privacy of domestic life, even among the most disadvantaged families; the different ethos and goals of a school and a social services department; divergent accountability and funding mechanisms and territorial boundaries; the ambiguity and breadth of the term 'child abuse'.

The wider context remains turbulent, exemplified by recent major reorganisations of agencies' legal responsibilities and funding mechanisms, such as the Community Care legislation, NHS Trusts, local management of schools and the general shift towards the purchaser–provider split, and still projected changes such as the reorganisation of local government and police boundaries. It seems questionable whether, for instance, pastoral care for troubled children in schools or the time of paediatricians awaiting court hearings will be adequately budgeted in an environment of competitive pricing and narrow goals.

The mandate to co-ordinate

It is, however, evident that the mandate to co-ordinate has powerfully conditioned the professional handling of child protection in Britain over the last twenty years, despite the complexities analysed in organisation theory and revealed in numerous theoretical and empirical texts on the phenomena of child abuse and practitioners' interventions. The weight of government guidance has reflected the politically high profile of the problem of child abuse and exceeds that given in other spheres of professional overlap such as mental health or the care of elderly and disabled people. There has been an emphasis on bureaucratic procedures relating to the identification and registration of abused children.

Five main mechanisms have developed since 1974.

1. *The Child Protection Register* This is generally maintained by the social services department but in some localities this is done by the NSPCC. It identifies children who are deemed to have been abused and since 1991 is restricted to those for whom a protection plan is necessary.
2. *The Interdisciplinary Child Protection Conference* This is generally convened and chaired by social services staff but in some localities by the NSPCC. It determines whether a child should be placed on the register. When necessary, it considers major changes of plan and periodically reviews progress.
3. *The Area Child Protection Committee* This has local policy-monitoring and training responsibilities, formulates local interagency guidelines and identifies 'significant issues arising from the handling of cases and reports from inquiries' (DOH 1991, p. 6). Despite its steadily increasing nominal responsibilities, this remains a constitutionally weak body which depends on the goodwill and funding of its diverse member agencies.
4. *The core group* This is a more recent formulation in recognition of the need for an ongoing forum where the practitioners most closely involved with an individual case discuss their inputs and case developments.
5. *The key worker* This is a social worker, generally from the social services department, who should be the focal point for all relevant information concerning an individual case and is responsible for maintaining the information network for that case.

Working Together and related official guidance are prescriptive about the need for both medical and social evaluation of all suspected cases of abuse and about the necessity to seek police background information and possibly also their investigative skills. The guidance is also categoric about the primacy of the child's welfare in eah case over other possibly conflicting agency goals such as prosecution of abusers. However, only recently has the official literature given a modest amount of attention to the skill content required by the various professions for effective intervention and successful long-term outcomes for the children concerned.

Recent government research has also been investigating a range of issues regarding children's and families' experience of interventions. Nevertheless, because child abuse is a term covering a very wide and disputed range of interpersonal phenomena, it is difficult to develop case management protocols or standards susceptible to professional audit, and it is still fair to say that more official scrutiny is given to procedural matters than to preventive or therapeutic effectiveness.

The first government circular was promulgated jointly by the Home Office, Ministry of Health and Ministry of Education in 1950, regarding *Children Ill-treated or Neglected in their Own Homes* (Home Office *et al.*, 1950). In fact, the occasional inter-agency case conferences, called by the Children's Departments to co-ordinate professional interventions with so-called 'problem families', were less preoccupied with procedural questions within the resource and skill constraints of the times, and more orientated towards effective case management.

It was, however, the death of Maria Colwell and the publication of the official Inquiry Report (1974) that caused a major seismic shock, arousing British consciousness to the issue of child abuse. Media reaction was intense and politicians and the social work profession were deeply affected. Subsequent inquiries into other child abuse tragedies drew attention, like the Maria Colwell Report, to failures of perception and of communication between a range of workers and agencies about the condition of the children concerned. Such inquiries dealt retrospectively with atypical cases and have revealed little interest in or ability to consider a range of wider issues that might constrain or facilitate effective handling of those particular cases, let alone of the generality of children deemed at risk at the time (Hallett, 1989).

The role of the social worker

Social workers have been the primary targets of media criticism for their alleged failure to protect children and, more recently, for acting too quickly or forcefully. This is despite the fact that they depend on medical diagnosis and police investigation in many cases and on courts to adjudicate on the need for compulsory interventions. Also, the vast majority of registered children have uneventful and apparently successful careers through the system. (Approximately 40 000 children were on child protection registers at any one time in the late 1980s and early 1990s.) Social workers remained the focus of criticism until the Cleveland affair over the newly prominent issue of sexual abuse also brought paediatricians and the police into contention (Cleveland Report, 1988).

In response to these pressures, from 1974 onwards central government guidance and local agency procedures have become more and more specific about the conduct of child protection registers, criteria for entering the names of individual children as 'abused' or 'at risk' and about mechanisms for exchanging information between workers (Birchall, 1989; Hallett and Birchall, 1992).

Interprofessional co-operation in this field is characterised by a greater public and political sensitivity than in many other overlapping fields of medical and social care. It is also made more complex for all participants by the range of agencies concerned but particularly by issues of social control, crime and police involvement. As Parton and Parton (1989) argue, social workers are often centrally concerned with negotiating the legal boundaries between the rights and responsibilities of the state and those of the family in the upbringing and care of their children. Social services departments hold the primary legal responsibility for investigating and evaluating suspicions of child maltreatment and seeking legal safeguards for the children as necessary. While the NSPCC and the police also have similar powers of immediate intervention, only the social services department has the function of arranging ongoing support and protection, whether at home or in care.

The theoretical literature, a number of empirical studies and professional experience all suggest that the combination of therapeutic care and social control is difficult, even though it may be desirable. No other agency has this specific combination of responsibilities which epitomises social work. Other professions such as doctors, health visitors and teachers may be reluctant to breach confidentiality and involve themselves with 'policing families' even though, as mentioned above, social workers frequently need their information and expertise in diagnosis and evaluation.

Interprofessional work: an empirical study

Many specific empirical studies in the USA have investigated, for instance, physicians' and teachers' reporting behaviour or uncovered antagonistic values and incompatible practices between police and social workers. Little empirical work had been done in the UK but Hallett and Stevenson (1980), Hilgendorf (1981), Dingwall *et al.* (1983), Corby (1987) and Wattam (undated) also reveal tensions in the British system. There are recurring complaints in Inquiry Reports about failures of communication and co-ordination. A rhetoric of commitment to co-operation in child protection exists, but there are numerous evident sources of conflict. Such is the background to the large research project reported below.

In addition to the literature review already cited, two field work phases between 1990 and 1992 were used to investigate aspects of interprofessional co-operation in the UK. The first (Birchall, 1992) comprised a postal survey of a stratified random sample of 339 workers in six professions: social workers, health visitors, primary school teachers, police specialists, general practitioners and paediatric doctors. It had been hoped to include local authority lawyers, a small but sometimes crucial element in the system, but they proved impossible to recruit. Individuals might or might not have had direct experience of cases but the questionnaire addressed their general experience and perceptions of the child protection system as regards work with children and families at the individual case level. The professions were chosen because they appeared from the literature and experience to be important sectors of the child protection system, although many others could have been embraced if resources had allowed. The last phase (Hallett, 1993) was a more qualitative investigation by means of a case records study and interviews with workers actually involved in a random series of recent cases. Thus it covered a somewhat wider range of professions which sometimes, rather than routinely, become involved.

Together the studies covered five areas in the north of England, selected to embrace a range of socio-demographic and organisational variables. The focal questions of the postal survey were:

- What experience of child protection work do the respondents have?
- How convergent or otherwise are respondents' perceptions of cases?
- What are their perceptions and evaluations of the local child protection system?
- Can the local network be mapped?
- What appear to be the most important factors influencing the above?
- What interpretations can be offered for the relationships discovered?
- What are the implications of the findings for policy and practice?

In the qualitative study, similar factual data was collected about the respondents and the semi-structured interviews and supplementary questionnaire also covered parallel fields.

The overall response rate to the postal survey was 60 per cent, varying from 81 per cent among health visitors to 38 per cent among general practitioners. Thus, the deliberate sampling bias towards the more involved professions was accentuated by the varying response rates. The response rate in the interview sample was extremely high (97 per cent) and, by definition, they were respondents with immediate involvement in cases. There were no significant variations between areas in either the personal variables or in respondents' exposure or attitudes to child protection work. Only a few questions showed inter-area variations, for instance different recourse to the NSPCC or community medical officers indicated varying local resources, but not among the core professions in the network.

Discrepancies in personal characteristics and status factors are often cited as sources of conflict and misunderstanding between collaborators. The stereotypes of young, trendy and constantly changing social workers, which can adversely affect interprofessional co-operation, are to some extent refuted by the data. Although their mobility is greater than among general practitioners or paediatric consultants, for instance, it is not a marked feature in these localities and is less than among the police or junior doctors. The data also suggest that health visitors and social workers tend to be recruited at a more mature age than the other professions. Not surprisingly, paediatric staff show the clearest differentiation of rank by age.

As expected, most doctors are men, while almost all health visitors and more social workers, police specialists and primary school teachers are women. Throughout the professions, men are disproportionately represented in the senior ranks. Educational levels vary markedly between the professions, with most doctors having postgraduate qualifications; social workers are evenly divided between non-graduates and postgraduates; less than half the teachers and few of the health visitors are graduates; none of the police in this sample have qualifications other than in-service police training.

The resulting data represent the views of staff whose personal characteristics are typical of the people in the network but, because of the sampling frames and the bias in response rates, respondents have more than average experience and interest in the practice of child protection. Taken together, the low participation rates of general practitioners and teachers and the number of 'don't knows' from those who did respond clearly indicate how peripheral child abuse is to the everyday world of these two large professional groups.

Main findings of the survey

Key professions

The general patterns of answers indicated that the key professions had been identified and incorporated in the survey design. They appear to be:

- general practitioners
- health visitors
- paediatricians
- police
- social workers
- teachers.

It is also evident that the above are not all equally involved and that some other professions are sometimes involved. The system appears to comprise five tiers, as shown in the following table.

Table 6.1 *The five-tier structure of the child protection system*

Tier	*Professions concerned*
Key worker	Social worker
Investigative professions	Social worker, paediatrician, police
Front line agencies	Schools, health visitors, general practitioners, social workers (in many cases)
Peripheral contact professions	School nurses, education welfare officers, community medical officers
Case-specific professions	Lawyers, psychiatrists, and many others

Social workers have many more contacts than any other group with the rest of the network. Health visitors emerge as a crucial link in the

mesh of front-line observation and support services in which teachers and general practitioners normally and social workers sometimes go about their business. However, individual teachers and
general practitioners were rarely involved in cases; their relative
prominence in the network is due to the size of their professions and
their universal coverage of the population. Fewer health visitors,
with a similar universal coverage, were individually much more
engaged in child protection activities than these other front-line
professions. As far as this research could reveal, the psychotherapeutic professions and probation were little involved.

Structural issues

The detailed findings can be broadly classified into structural, procedural and case issues, and some of the more important ones are
sketched below. While it is important to note that there were varied
opinions within each professional group on almost all topics, profession was the main independent variable correlating with almost all
divergences of view. However, profession and experiential factors
frequently overlapped.

Experience

Experience of child protection work varied widely between the
professions, although over four-fifths of the survey respondents had
been involved to at least a minimal degree in a case in the preceding
year. The range was from no cases in many teachers' whole working
life to a senior police co-ordinator's contact with over 2000 cases
within the year; however, the largest number (44 per cent) had been
engaged in fewer than ten cases. Involvement in child protection
conferences similarly varies widely. Social workers, the police and
paediatricians clearly emerge as the core professions in the child
protection network. The police have an exceptionally heavy
throughput of cases but they and paediatricians are generally only
briefly involved. Health visitors occupy an intermediate position but
each general practitioner and teacher is rarely involved.

Specific training either in handling child abuse cases or in the
processes of interprofessional co-operation is extremely limited. Although most practitioners directly involved in the case sample had
some such training, half the survey sample have had none what-
soever and very few have more than a fortnight. Most of the surveyed social workers, health visitors, police and paediatric
consultants have some, but very few teachers, general practitioners

or junior doctors have any. For most participants, some of this training has been on an interdisciplinary basis but the experience is very narrow for most. The commonest pairing is of social workers and police, although paediatricians, health visitors and social workers have frequently shared. Otherwise, there is a tendency for the medical professions to train together rather than with broader groups.

Most of those concerned found such training a positive experience but there is some evidence that different professions seek and value different aspects of it, with teachers most appreciative of new knowledge, health visitors and the police highlighting the importance of discovering others' roles and skills and social workers most concerned about developing co-operative processes.

Perceptions of interprofessional contacts

The data about contact patterns arose from case vignettes in the survey and is supported by data from the case study. In addition, respondents' perceptions of twelve professions sometimes involved in the child protection network were explored through scaled questions. These covered four factors: the ease of co-operating with them, the clarity and importance of their roles and their performance in this field. A very large majority claimed some experience, however limited, of most of the professions named, the lowest response being 55 per cent in relation to lawyers. There were, however, significant numbers of general practitioners and teachers who indicated no relevant experience overall or in relation to specific others; almost everyone else had a wide range of contacts. These questions gave further evidence of the tiered structure indicated above. It was interesting that some experience of the core professions was nearly as prevalent as experience of the front-line professions. However, the core professions themselves, with health visitors, formed the densest network of interactions.

The bulk of substantive responses to all professions rated them fairly positively on all factors but there are some marked variations. Opinions about social workers are split, with sizeable minorities finding them either very easy or difficult to work with. School nurses and health visitors are reported to be particularly easy and the balance of opinion about the police is favourable, although teachers and general practitioners showed a rather guarded attitude towards them through their responses to the long vignettes.

There is widespread dissatisfaction or uncertainty regarding general practitioners' contribution to child protection on all four factors. All the medical professions are found difficult more often than others and rated as very difficult by significant minorities. However, a quarter of respondents find working with paediatricians very easy. Generally, doctors find it easier to work with social workers and health visitors than vice versa, and this marked imbalance in the collaborative relationship is familiar in the literature.

A large majority feel very or fairly clear about the role of the core professions but a worrying number, particularly of teachers, only feel fairly clear about social workers. As befits their co-ordinating role, social workers are the most likely to recognise the importance of a wider range of other professions, although few respondents rate any profession's contribution as unimportant. There is a high consensus on the essential role of social workers but considerable confusion about the role of teachers, health visitors and general practitioners, not least among themselves. That the front-line professions are generally deemed as important as the investigative professions is a welcome indication that most members of the network have a wider view of child protection than the merely forensic.

Fewer people feel able to comment on others' performance of their roles, apparently due to their limited experience or lack of feedback, but the bulk of responses deem that others fulfilled their functions fairly well. Sizeable minorities think the core professions and health visitors perform very well. Social workers were most often critical, particularly of doctors, but they thought highly of the police. Generally, greater experience increased people's scepticism about other groups' role performance but this was not so concerning paediatricians. In their case, interview data showed that the attitudes or interests of individual doctors were particularly influential over others' evaluations.

A basic finding was that the need for co-operation was very widely accepted by active members of the network. It appears that mandated co-ordination has had a major impact on people's perceptions and practice and that the policy implementation gap has been quite effectively bridged. Social services departments' lead role in the system was no longer in contention; there was no hint of the conflict between social services and paediatricians over who should chair child protection conferences that Dingwall *et al.* (1983) observed ten years ago. Objections to police involvement were no longer evident on many respondents' agenda.

Constraints on interprofessional work

Most people felt the system worked 'rather well' and that relationships were generally 'rather good'. Only one-fifth believe interprofessional co-ordination works 'very well' in the assessment phase and over a quarter consider ongoing co-ordination is poor. While there was no evidence of major structural conflict, the survey showed and the interview sample sharply illustrated a number of expected issues. There was concern and sadness, rather than conflict, among many professions that resource constraints prevented co-operative services which they perceived as appropriate. The many real obstacles to co-operation ranged from conflicting priorities in different agencies and other professional tensions to shortage of time.

For instance, early referrals to social workers for preventive work were impossible and ready admission of children to paediatric wards for a non-stigmatising assessment increasingly unlikely. Joint police – social work interviews were often not conducted responsively at the child's pace but under acute pressures, which related to the very rapid and heavy case turnover of the police and also revealed significant tensions about whose skills and purposes should dominate. Keeping in touch with the numerous and frequently changing staff in the network is a particular problem for social workers and health visitors, a large number of main grade staff in these two less prestigious professions being handicapped by prosaic problems like shortage of secretarial support and telephones. It should be a matter of great concern that the key worker in particular is deprived of the tools for communication and recording.

The following quotation describing one social worker's encounters with some paediatricians vividly illuminates several issues of status conflict, role responsibilities and interpersonal variability:

> We sometimes have to say to them 'I need to know from you categorically, is this consistent or is it not consistent? Does it fit or doesn't it fit? And you're going to need to tell me that now. You know we can't be saying oh it could be, or, it couldn't be, and I need you to stick with that – what you're telling me now is what's going to be in your report because that is also very important.' I suppose they see me as a very mouthy person who is continually saying 'I want to see you, it's important, that's what I'm looking for' and I don't know actually how they perceive that, not only as men, there's an age differential as well, a gender differential and there's also a professional differential that they are consultant paediatricians and I am a social worker.

Thus, beside the manifest general goodwill, there are many structural frictions, imperfect communications and interpersonal disagreements. There are no data to suggest that the breakdowns of perception or co-operation held to account in the occasional tragic inquiry cases that have so conditioned public opinion are in any way characteristic of the system. On the contrary, maybe both the system and most registered families are robust enough to survive these frictions and the causes of catastrophe should be sought elsewhere.

Specific proposals for improvement were less frequent than general assertions that 'communication' was crucial. Social workers and health visitors indicated most awareness of relevant issues and perhaps most interest in making the network function. These findings would appear to reflect the social worker's official responsibility as key worker and the role that health visitors actually occupy as a crucial link between the frontline agencies and the child protection services.

Procedural issues

There was a broad acceptance of the importance of co-ordination, practically among the professionals involved in the qualitative case study and at least theoretically among the more diffuse survey respondents. However, the larger sample's awareness and use of the child protection machinery appear as variable as their reactions to cases.

Regarding the Area Child Protection Committee guidelines, the case study sample respondents were quite positive about their realism and helpfulness. In contrast, various data from the survey suggest that compliance among the potential network is often poor. While half the latter sample claim that they fully adhere to the guidelines in all cases, knowledge of their contents proved to vary widely.

Almost all social workers have their own copy and refer to it frequently but at the other extreme many general practitioners and teachers would not know where to find one. A significant minority believe they would have to go to another building to see a copy. A number of people in all professions doubt the relevance and realism of the guidelines, either because they are busy, or because cases vary in ways that procedures cannot encompass. Some professions find the procedures more helpful than others. Social workers and health visitors are the most appreciative of the guidelines and make the most complaints about others' serious lapses. In contrast, paediatricians are the most sceptical about their value. General practitioners most often complain that they have been poorly publicised while social workers more often believe they are poorly enforced in other agencies.

The general picture regarding workers' use of written communications gives grounds for concern. Both the survey and the case study showed that many exchanges apparently go unrecorded even on people's own case notes. Although direct cues led most survey respondents to say they would check the child protection register, the case study showed the majority of enquiries to come from social workers. Both sources show that even among social workers few see it as a dynamic and important information resource.

Respondents appear unclear about the circumstances in which a child protection conference should be sought and most appear to leave to social services staff not only the convening but also the proposal of a conference. Yet other data in the survey and some of the literature indicate that social workers are less likely to seek a conference at the same thresholds and that other agencies are sometimes dissatisfied with the lack of response to their concerns. Among the active minority, paediatricians most frequently propose a conference in these circumstances, but general practitioners are also prominent – surprisingly, in view of their low profile in the conference system.

To a very large extent, participants consider conferences useful to themselves, particularly in clarifying professional assessments, but also in serving a number of other purposes. There appears to be much common ground about appropriate conference attenders but there were disagreements about the appropriate mix of ranks. The particular choices are in line with the multilayered pattern of frontline, core and peripheral agencies and sub-systems already identified. The most frequent dissatisfaction is about the absence of general practitioners, who report extreme difficulty in attending despite their infrequent involvement in cases. Other doctors, although nominated less frequently, are wanted conspicuously more often than expected. Many other workers with a heavy burden of cases or of conference attendance also find it problematic but appear more willing to prioritise their attendance. There is a tendency for the different professions to say their lot would be eased if only the conference would meet on their premises.

Frequent tension is acknowledged by a significant number of respondents on matters of professional role, beliefs and values, and also around the interpretation and application of the procedural guidelines to particular cases. However, more interprofessional training correlates with a higher appreciation of the contribution of conferences to case management and more confidence that disputes are manageable. Those with such training also strongly disagree with the notion that they waste time.

Nevertheless, most respondents feel conferences could be improved. The leading proposals were for better attendance by crucial people and for the circulation of prior written information. Doctors emerge as more concerned about timetabling, smaller and shorter meetings but much less concerned than social workers about absentees. Social workers make most suggestions about improving the administration of meetings, and it may be that the specifics they suggest would go at least part way to meeting the doctors' superficially different preoccupations. Despite increasing pressure from official policy-makers, there is no consensus in this study about the attendance of parents or children; the conflicting opinions crosscut professions and personal views.

In parallel with their esteem for the procedural guidelines and arguably for the same structural reasons, health visitors have the highest opinion of conferences while general practitioners are the most guarded on many points. However, social workers are the most sceptical about conferences' capacity for managing professional anxieties and they perceive most role conflict between workers. These negative views seem likely to reflect their difficult role of 'managing from below' (Weightman, 1988).

Discrepant responses to cases

In contrast to those in the interview sample who appeared satisfied that referrals to the child protection system were generally pitched at the right level, the survey found considerable uncertainty among the broader sample of potential identifiers and referral agents about the classification and management of ambiguous vignettes of possible maltreatment. A very large majority of respondents proposed some intervention and also some interagency contact about all the vignettes. Within these broad outlines, however, there were many differences. People's views on appropriate interventions varied, with different contact networks being identified. Some would refer such cases directly into the child protection, system but there was a tendency for teachers and general practitioners to retain cases within their medical or educational networks or for teachers to attempt to support such cases themselves.

Readiness to conceptualise a situation as child abuse resulted in advocacy of a more investigative approach; this was not consistently related to people's professional locus but rather more to greater experience of child protection. Generally, people appeared more anxious, intrusive and confrontational with a story of possible sexual abuse and with a story involving a black family than when the same data were presented without the family's race being specified.

Most agreed that the names of all the children in the vignettes should be placed on the child protection register but very few respondents favoured removal from home for any of them. Many people made alternative and sometimes contradictory recommendations for them, revealing the genuine difficulties of the job. On the whole, the higher up the tariff of options, the more people of all ranks and professions said they did not know what to propose. Social workers and others with much relevant experience most frequently advocated supporting them at home on a voluntary footing. Despite or perhaps because of their limited experience, general practitioners predominated among the small number seeking their removal from home.

As in Giovannoni and Becerra (1979), there were also significant variations in the severity rating given to a series of brief vignettes. Cases in the physical and sexual abuse categories are evidently rated more severely than neglect or emotional abuse, by all the professions. Total interprofessional consensus in ratings occurred in only the most severe minority of cases. The coalitions of view vary from case to case but most disagreements arose between health visitors who rate cases most severely and social workers who rate them least severely. Teachers' tendency to rate cases severely also distinguishes them significantly from social workers. General practitioners, paediatricians and, perhaps more surprisingly, the police showed no significant divergences in ratings. Paediatricians revealed individually rather varied but corporately median ratings.

The divergent evaluations of social workers, health visitors and teachers are likely to cause friction or concern in the front line supporting families, as evidenced in some of the interview data. Social workers will react to;

> a great big bruise on Jonathan's leg [but] we have nine classes and could have five families that we are quite desperately worried about in each class . . . I can appreciate their side, you know, they've got such a large area to cover.

Nevertheless, it may be reassuring that there are relatively few divergences in severity ratings between the core investigative professions.

The literature is divided about whether it is more effective to start interventions with parents on the basis of supportive acceptance by the professionals, or to take an approach which stresses parental acceptance of responsibility, or whether it is possible to combine them. Such a philosophical rift would be likely to cause conflict between workers and may affect their attitudes to referral into the child protection system. While many people in all professions appear to have complex and probably confused attitudes, admitting a variety of contingent factors which would affect their choice of approach, probing showed that the core professions were rather more likely to dismiss the relevance of situational factors than the front-line professions. This attitudinal difference between the core and front-line professions is far from clear-cut, but more child protection training was correlated with less attention to contingent factors. There is also greater homogeneity between and within the professions in advocating a confrontational approach to cases of sexual abuse. Overall, however, there were marked variations which appeared to derive from individual as well as professional values.

It is evident that almost all co-operation and co-ordination comprises the exchange of information. Social workers are the most likely target of simple referrals, while teachers and general practitioners are more often involved in information exchanges than other transactions. When they are involved, paediatricians are the target of referrals and a source of advice. They also generally make most use of external resources. In general, people reported more intentions to exchange information immediately to hand than to maintain a collaborative relationship.

Only the police and social workers are doing any significant amounts of 'hands on' joint work. This confirms the continuing primacy of the forensic task and continuing underdevelopment of planned, interdisciplinary therapeutic interventions with the children or their families of the sort occasionally mentioned in the literature.

Interdisciplinary collaboration

The limited scope and spread of relevant training and the evidently varying commitment of the different professions to interdisciplinary training is a matter for concern. Given the evidence of difficulties in collaboration between doctors and others and the crucial role of paediatricians, it seems particularly regrettable that junior doctors get no interdisciplinary preparation for the moment when they will dive into the system from a very high board. The profound questions of gender, educational and organisational status differentials are difficult to overcome.

The gap between doctors' views of and compliance with the procedures and those of social workers and health visitors indicates the continuing salience of status and power. The former can apparently afford to be less compliant, being less susceptible to agency or public sanction and perceiving themselves to be less in need of the others' inputs to their case management. On the other hand, the social workers and health visitors are organisationally more vulnerable and also probably more reliant on the procedures in their efforts to induce co-operation from other members of the network. While it might be possible for Area Child Protection Committees to be more active in promulgating the guidelines, it is more difficult to resolve the problem of enforcement among such diverse organisational structures.

Case conferences were generally valued, although several criticisms and suggestions for their better organisation were voiced. Some disagreements highlight ambiguities and dilemmas about the complex functions of conferences and suggest that the emergence of the core group meeting is an important development for the hands-on collaborators.

The literature, survey data and interviews suggest a distance between social workers and general practitioners in the arena of child protection, which may be disturbing in view of the latter's presumed role as primary identifiers of abused children. The case study data showed that general practitioners only appeared as referring agents when mothers themselves had told them directly about such situations. The survey suggests that there are sub-systems around the medical centre and also the school. While these probably contain many cases appropriately, some data suggest that professional proximity rather than the needs of the case may sometimes influence the choice of relationships. Thus, some communication chains may be unduly stretched and insecure, for instance, from class teacher to head to school nurse to health visitor to social worker. It is thus possible that the sub-systems may sometimes inappropriately divert cases from child protection investigation. Health visitors appear to have a critical role as a fulcrum between those sub-systems and the sphere of child protection in which social workers, the police and paediatricians have very specific roles.

Although anxiety was an evident factor in people's reaction to child protection work and there were indications that people often turned to external colleagues for advice and support, sometimes in preference to their own management, the patterns and content of communication suggest that the professional network is not a 'team' that can give emotional support to the practitioners. If mutual trust and collaborative relationships depend considerably on proximity, the essential partners must, as the literature argues (Hallett and Birchall, 1992, chs 11 and 14), create and be given the opportunity to invest time with one another and in joint training.

The lack of consensus about the cases deemed less severe must cause problems in establishing a baseline for protective intervention, particularly among front-line workers or in cases of neglect and emotional abuse. There is some support for the stereotypical view of overanxious health visitors and teachers pressing impassive social workers who will not be moved. Social workers and health visitors are the two professions most frequently interweaving their continuing support and observation of the same troubled families and, if teachers' pastoral role were exploited more systematically, similar tensions could become more obvious.

Uncertainties and conflicting responses throughout the vignette sequences are mirrored in the fact that only a minority expect consensus to be easily achieved in a conference dealing with such case material. Whereas teachers showed most inclination to say they did not know what to recommend at a conference, social workers were most and doctors least likely to expect to be disagreed with. Despite social workers' greater experience and primary responsibility for the future of the case, the conflicts between them and doctors about future management appear to arise more often from discrepancies of status and organisational structure than from disputes about the initial severity ratings they give to cases.

General conclusions

There is a broad acceptance of the need for interprofessional co-operation in this field and a general perception that the system works 'fairly well'. However, most of the interagency activity comprises exchanges of information in the early stages of identification and assessment and there is very little evidence of close, continuing collaboration. How much 'hands-on' collaboration is desirable and between whom, are matters that may emerge more clearly as the experience of core groups builds up, even though resource constraints on effective intervention are strongly evident.

Despite the generally favourable attitudes to co-ordination, there are many divergences in people's responses which confirm that it is often problematic.

Profession is the factor that most affects perceptions and actions in dealing with abused children and their families, not only in the obvious sense of fulfilling a task specific to the person's job but more pervasively in influencing the worker's perception of a case, of the way it should be handled, of the appropriate network to engage with and of his or her place in that network. Clearly, personal judgments and values are also significant factors in individuals' decisions and choices in case management in child protection and there are few points on which there is a massive consensus either between the professions or within each group. However, there are consistencies in the data which are best expressed as more or less likely postures.

A hypothesis proven unfounded was that three contrasting locations might reveal discrepant local policies and professional and agency cultures which would significantly affect people's decisions about cases. This was not so, and the respondent's locality also had surprisingly little correlation with perceptions of policy and co-ordinating machinery. The local guidelines showed many similarities. It appears that a fairly uniform national culture and a common procedural framework of working together has developed over recent years, although discrepancies between individuals and professions evidently remain.

Despite their salience to some issues in the literature, gender, age and child-rearing experience correlate with almost none of the case perceptions in this study. However, as one would expect from the literature on gender and on the sociology of the professions, gender appears to be a pertinent factor in some aspects of interprofessional relationships, but it is entwined with a whole bundle of status factors that are associated with different professional roles.

There were insufficient respondents from ethnic minority groups to test the effect of ethnicity in interprofessional relationships but it was significant and troubling that people reacted more suspiciously and anxiously, perhaps harshly, to the black variant of a vignette than to the one of unspecified race. The greater readiness to label the case as suspected abuse, fewer proposals of direct help and more reference to social work agencies than to paediatric help, all suggest a process of stigmatisation. These findings, of considerable significance for black families, are important issues for the child protection system and for strategies to combat racism in the health and welfare services.

Widespread differences of opinion about starting work with families from a more confrontational or supportive approach are only partly influenced by professional orientation or role; they also appear quite strongly to reflect personal value systems. They must remain powerful dynamics, whether hidden or openly-debated, in the activities of any group of workers either within a single agency or across different disciplines.

As a general conclusion, the interactions proposed in response to the vignettes appear partly to reflect case needs and professional functions but some may have more to do with easy access or status than with the functions and skills of those concerned.

These many differences in approach to cases reveal the lack of any established technical consensus within or across the professions as to the best means of handling such situations. That there is a complex cross-cutting of respondents' tasks and roles and varied perceptions in relation to different cases, which then lead to different proposals, is not a surprising finding – but it does mean that much co-operative activity in the child protection network is situationally specific, probably extremely difficult for the practitioners to articulate into generalised rules and certainly difficult to conceptualise theoretically.

Some of the discrepancies are no doubt inherent in the different personal and cultural values of each individual in this society and Kempe and Helfer's (1972) observation on the importance of essentially different people providing interpersonal data for the assessment remains pertinent. However, it is worth considering whether more interprofessional training and joint rating exercises, backed up by some common education in child development, could reduce the differences.

Most of the discussion has therefore related to individual and professional variations in perception and judgements and their likely impact on co-operative relationships. While such differences are frequent, they seem better categorised as frictions than breakdowns in the process of co-operation. However, it is possible that the large proportion of non-respondent general practitioners and smaller but significant number of paediatric refusers conceal a more disaffected attitude.

Significant frictions are evident between social workers and doctors but surprisingly absent between social workers and the police. They are likely to be of greater concern when they arise with paediatricians than other doctors because of the need for close co-operation within the core group. Some differences are explicable in terms of professional task or agency function and may often be unproblematic. Others, where different workers' tasks and priorities may clash, may be sources of conflict: these indicate individual opinions in a contentious and uncertain sphere of work or role confusion within and between the professions, any of which may lead to unrealistic or incompatible expectations of what individuals will or should do.

When the cogs of the machine begin to grate for any of these reasons and discrepant expectations arise, then it is likely that political factors of power and status and resource dependency will come into play and domain conflicts may also emerge. Although less than in earlier accounts, these still appear significant between social workers and paediatricians, illustrated in their different expectations regarding disagreements in conference which indicate that professional status is still an important influence. Social workers are relatively highly-educated and not younger than other professionals, but as key workers they are frequently negotiating with senior staff in other agencies. It is well recognised that a number of status factors – professional prestige, rank, educational level, frequently male gender – combine in the person of the consultant paediatrician. When these also coincide with greater age and local experience, as they tend to, power imbalances are likely in the network.

Such factors are difficult to uncover and were not often overtly acknowledged in the interviews or the survey but, as one would expect from the literature, are strongly suggested by some of the response patterns. This suggests that action plans will still be to a large extent the outcome of the fundamentally moral and political processes of interprofessional negotiation that Dingwall *et al.* (1983) analysed.

References

Aldrich, H. E. (1972), 'An Organisational-Environment Perspective on Co-operation and Conflict between Organisations in the Manpower and Training System', in A. Neghandi (ed.), *Interorganisation Theory*. (Englewood Cliffs, N. J.: Prentice Hall).

Aldrich, H. E. (1976), 'Resource Dependence and Interorganisational Relations', in *Administration and Society*, no. 7, pp. 419–54.

Aldrich, H. E. (1979), *Organisations and Environments* (Englewood Cliffs, N. J.: Prentice Hall).

Benson, J. K. (1975), 'The Interorganisational Network as a Political Economy', *Administrative Science Quarterly*, no. 20, pp. 229–49.

Birchall, E. (1989), 'The Frequency of Child Abuse – what do we really know?', in O. Stevenson (ed.), *Child Abuse: Public Policy and Professional Practice* (Hemel Hempstead: Harvester Wheatsheaf).

Birchall, E. (1992), *Working Together in Child Protection: Report of Phase Two, a Survey of the Experience and Perceptions of Six Key Professions* (Stirling: University of Stirling).

Christopherson, J. (1989), 'European Child Abuse Management Systems', in Olive Stevenson (ed.), *Child Abuse: Public Policy and Professional Practice* (Hemel Hempstead: Harvester Wheatsheaf).

Cleveland Report (1988), *Report of the Inquiry into Child Abuse in Cleveland 1987*, Cmnd. 412 (London: HMSO).

Colwell Report (1974), *Report of the Committee of Inquiry into the Care and Supervision provided in relation to Maria Colwell* (Chair: T.G. Field-Fisher) (London: HMSO).

Corby, B. (1987), *Working with Child Abuse* (Milton Keynes: Open University Press).

Dale, P., Davies, M., Morrison, T. and Waters, J. (1986), *Dangerous Families: Assessment and Treatment of Child Abuse* (London: Tavistock).

Department of Health (1988), *Protecting Children: a guide for social workers undertaking a comprehensive assessment* (London: HMSO).

Department of Health (1991), *Working Together under the Children Act 1989: a Guide to Arrangements for Inter-Agency Co- operation for the Protection of Children from Abuse* (London: HMSO).

Department of Health and Social Security (1973), *Report of the Tunbridge Wells Study Group* (London: DHSS).

Dingwall, R., Eekelaar, J. and Murray, T. (1983), *The Protection of Children: State Intervention and Family Life* (Oxford: Blackwell).

Giovannoni, J. M. and Becerra, R. M. (1979), *Defining Child Abuse* (New York: Free Press).

Hallett, C. (1989), 'Child Abuse Inquiries and Public Policy', in O. Stevenson (ed.), *Child Abuse: Public Policy and Professional Practice* (Hemel Hempstead: Harvester Wheatsheaf).

Hallett, C. (1993), *Working Together in Child Protection: Report of Phase Three, a Case Study of Coordination Policies and Practices* (Stirling: University of Stirling).

Hallett, C. and Birchall, E. (1992), *Coordination and Child Protection: a Review of the Literature* (Edinburgh: HMSO).

Hallett, C. and Stevenson, O. (1980), *Child Abuse: Aspects of Interprofessional Cooperation* (London: Allen & Unwin).

Hauf, K. (1978), 'Introduction', in K. Hauf and F. W. Scharpf (eds), *Interorganisational Policy-making: Limits to Co- ordination and Central Control* (London and Beverly Hills: Sage).

Hilgendorf, L. (1981), *Social Workers and Solicitors in Child Care Cases* (London: HMSO).

Home Office, Ministry of Health and Ministry of Education (1950), *Children Ill-treated or Neglected in their own Homes* (London: HMSO).

Kempe, C. H., Silverman, F. N., Steele, B. F., Droegmueller, W. and Silver, H. K. (1962), 'The Battered Child Syndrome', *Journal of the American Medical Association*, 181, pp. 17–22.

Kempe, C. H. and Helfer, R. E. (eds) (1972), *Helping the Battered Child and his Family* (Philadelphia: Lippincott and Co.).

Levine, S. and White, P. E. (1961), 'Exchange as a Conceptual Framework for the Study of Interorganisational Relationships', *Administrative Science Quarterly*, 5, pp. 583–601.

Parton, C. and Parton, N. (1989), 'Child Protection, the Law and Dangerousness', in O. Stevenson (ed.), *Child Abuse: Public Policy and Professional Practice* (Hemel Hempstead: Harvester Wheatsheaf).

Wattam, C. (undated), *Teachers' Experience with Children who have or may have been Sexually Abused,* (London: NSPCC).

Weightman, K. (1988), 'Managing from Below', *Social Work Today,* 29 September, pp. 16–17.

7 *Mental health services*

Roslyn Corney

Chapter summary

The author describes the multidisciplinary approach that is essential to the provision of high quality mental health services. The diversity of client needs means that more than one agency is involved. An overview of research in collaborative practice and an historical overview of service development supports the conclusion that co-ordinated services are better for mentally-ill people. Strategies for improving interprofessional and interagency work are discussed, especially in the context of primary health care teams.

The extent of illness and distress

In 1990 The Mental Health Foundation (MHF) indicated that approximately 6 million people in Britain suffer from some of mental illness or distress each year. Of these people, approximately 3.7 million were classified as severely ill (MHF, 1990). In the late 1980s it was estimated that there were 60,000 people resident in mental illness hospitals, which suggests that the majority of severely ill people are now resident outside hospital. Thus for most people care is provided in the community. For example, there were nearly 2 million outpatient attendances made each year to psychiatrists (Office of Health Economics [OHE], 1989). Other NHS and local authority services include psychiatric and social service day care, community clinics including community mental health centres, as well as home and clinic visits by community psychiatric nurses, psychologists and social workers. It has also been estimated that between 4 and 5 million people each year consult their general practitioners because of some kind of 'mental distress', most commonly depression and/or anxiety. To these figures can be added the number of contacts made by other members of the primary care team, such as practice nurses, health visitors and community nurses. Then there are the contacts with voluntary agencies and services associated with housing, income support and employment.

137

The extent of illness underlines the importance that should be attached to the effective delivery of mental health services. In future years, the need for services will increase with the rise in senile dementia brought about by an ageing population. This chapter will focus on adult services for the mentally ill and distressed. Provision for children, the elderly and those with learning disabilities will not be included.

The term 'mental illness'

There are major problems with the usage of the term 'mental illness'. There are many different groups of people suffering from some kind of mental distress and their needs for support and treatment vary. Careful consideration should be made before the term illness is applied, particularly for those conditions where no biological evidence of disorder has been found. There are also problems involved with the stigma attached to the label and with the fact that it can be used to justify the removal of an individual's civil rights. Another issue is that defining as ill individuals with symptoms of depression and anxiety (symptoms which the majority of us will experience during our lifetime) will medicalise these difficulties. This may lead to a more biological approach to treatment rather than helping clients in other ways such as attending to their social, practical and psychological needs.

Why is interprofessional collaboration necessary?

People with mental disùtress have a variety of needs which either accompany or are an outcome of the distress. This may include the need for suitable accommodation, employment and occupation, advice and practical help, education, social and leisure activities, income support and transport. They may need treatment for problems associated with physical ill-health. Their carers will also need to be supported in a number of ways.

This multiplicity of needs means that in most cases more than one service should be involved. There are variety of agencies relating to health, social services, employment and housing as well as the voluntary sector. As more people move from hospital to community care, continuity of care and co-ordination of services becomes even more vital. In the community, clients may be easily lost in the system or not picked up by the services sufficiently quickly (Langsley, 1975; Leff, 1993.)

Many of the problems preventing the effective delivery of services are due to poor communication between different professionals and different agencies. The responsibility for operating services in the community is fragmented between health authorities, local government, voluntary organisations and the private sector. Fragmentation is an inevitable consequence of a system with multiple agencies as well as a number of professionals who will often have varying objectives and viewpoints. These bodies have different styles, managers, priorities, structures and budgets.

A co-ordinated service requires effective communication between the different personnel involved in the care of any client and in the development of care plans – users and relatives should also be an integral part of this process. Effective communication systems need to be developed so that clients are not overlooked or lost to the system. This is particularly important in terms of the long-term and severely distressed client who may drop out of treatment. These clients are often not demanding or assertive and may not seek help on their own behalf unless others act as their advocates.

Evidence of poor collaboration – unmet need

A number of studies have shown that attending only to the psychiatric symptoms of clients while neglecting their other needs leads to poor overall client outcome. Professionals and helpers need to see clients in relation to their social and personal situation and to address the range of needs presented (Huxley *et al.*, 1990). This can often be only done if different agencies or professionals are involved and are working in collaboration.

A number of studies have indicated that in many cases, clients with severe distress have not received help to meet medical and social needs. A study by Pantellis and Taylor using the South Camden register, found that only 60 per cent of patients with a diagnosis of schizophrenia were in continuing contact with the psychiatric services (1988). Likewise Lee and Murray, studying a group of chronically ill patients, found that over half had lost contact with the psychiatric services (1988). Johnstone and colleagues (1984) interviewed 66 discharged patients and found that 27 per cent had no contact with any medical or social services. This study found that many informants had severe emotional, social and financial problems. Carers also had a number of unmet needs. The informants and relatives would have preferred a system where one person was the named key worker, aware of all the relevant details. The authors concluded that the services were limited in dealing with the multiple needs of those with severe and chronic illness.

Some studies have indicated that even those clients in close contact with services have many unmet needs. One analysis assessed the met and unmet needs of 145 people in long-term psychiatric day care (including day hospital and social service day centres). A typical member of the series was rated as having more than five types of clinical and social problem, each of which would require intervention by current professional standards (Brewin *et al.*, 1988; Brugha *et al.*, 1988). The study indicated that social service day centre attenders had over 1.5 times more clinical unmet needs than day hospital attenders and over twice as many unmet social needs.

Holloway (1991) also studied day care attenders. Staff at day centres often found difficulty in obtaining help for their clients from the hospital while hospital-based staff had little perception of what went on outside their own unit. The findings suggest that once a place in a day centre is found, input by other services such as the social work or the community psychiatric nursing service comes to an end or is markedly reduced. In general, there was little evidence of two-way regular communication or any attempts by community or psychiatric services to involve and work together with day centre staff on the development and implementation of a co-ordinated multi-agency treatment or rehabilitation plan.

Hoult (1986) indicated that more positive outcomes are reliant on comprehensive and continuous care. Components of care should include intensive initial help, patient and family involvement in planning, a case manager, practical help and a continuous 24-hour service which provides a rapid response in a crisis.

Collaboration with primary care

Ninety-eight per cent of the population defined as mentally ill are registered with their GP. Those with long-term and severe illness rely on their GP for ongoing psychiatric and medical help, and it seems inevitable that the role of the GP as the point of first contact will grow (Goldberg and Huxley, 1980; Corney, 1990).

In Great Britain, the extent of psychiatric morbidity presenting to primary care was first established in 1966. In a large-scale study of London general practices it was found that of 15,000 patients at risk in any twelve-month period, fourteen per cent consulted at least once for a condition diagnosed as entirely or largely psychiatric in nature (Shepherd *et al.*, 1966). Goldberg and Blackwell (1970) differentiated between the 'conspicuous' psychiatric morbidity detected by the general practitioner, and suggested that a further ten to twelve per cent went 'hidden' or unrecognised by the doctors. Similar studies conducted here (Skuse and Williams, 1984) and in the United States (Regier *et al.*, 1985) have suggested that approximately one-third of current attenders have some form of mental distress.

Previous studies have suggested that GPs have in general poor collaborative relationships with other non-medical agencies such as social services (Corney, 1980; Clare and Corney, 1982; Parsloe and Stevenson, 1980). Studies have also indicated that GPs are often not included in case discussions and treatment plans made by secondary care agencies (Thomas and Corney, 1993), and that hospital-based staff seldom attend case conferences outside the hospital (Dingwall, 1982).

The majority of doctors now work in group practices and employ receptionists, secretarial staff and practice nurses. Since the mid 1970s, the majority of health visitors and district nurses are either attached to general practices or liaising on a regular basis. GPs and other members of the primary care team (practice nurses, community nurses and health visitors) are in a good position to undertake preventive measures, as they are the professionals most likely to have ongoing contact with a number of high risk groups in the community, people suffering from bereavement, chronic illness, carers, women in the postnatal period and mothers with young children. Even as far back as the 1960s, Shepherd and colleagues suggested that 'the cardinal requirement for improvement of the mental health services . . . is not a large expansion of and proliferation of psychiatric agencies, but rather a strengthening of the family doctor in his therapeutic role, (Shepherd *et al.*, 1966). This was reiterated in the 1970s by the World Health Organization, which stated that the primary medical care team is the cornerstone of community psychiatry (WHO, 1973). An even stronger case can be made today for all mental health professionals and agencies to form close links and working relationships with general practitioners and other staff based in primary health care.

Evidence that co-ordinated services are better

Studies evaluating the work of mental health specialists in primary care have produced equivocal results in terms of clinical outcome.

Recent research conducted in Edinburgh found no clinical difference at sixteen weeks between mentally distressed clients (diagnosed with neurotic disorders) randomly allocated to one of four treatment groups: anti-depressants and psychiatrist care; cognitive behaviour therapy from a clinical psychologist; counselling and case work from a social worker; or normal GP treatment (Scott and Freeman, 1992). On the other hand, some studies have found more positive outcomes of primary care interventions by specialists, for example, three controlled trials of social worker effectiveness showed clinical improvement in the experimental group receiving additional social work help (Cooper *et al.*, 1975; Ross and Scott, 1985), although in one study this increased improvement only occurred in a subgroup of clients (Corney, 1984). Clinical psychologists have been shown to bring about recovery more quickly than occurs in control groups, even if the difference disappears at a longer-term follow-up (Robson *et al.*, 1984; Teasdale *et al.*, 1984). CPNs working in the home or practice with patients requiring follow-up were as effective as psychiatric outpatient care (Paykel *et al.*, 1982). Patients suffering from postnatal depression counselled by health visitors showed better outcome than those receiving routine GP care (Holden *et al.*, 1989). However, there is evident need for more research on whether integrated services perform much better than the present system in terms of client satisfaction, clinical improvement and social outcome.

The reasons for poor collaboration

The continued reliance on psychiatric hospitals and the underdevelopment of community facilities is bound up with the status and livelihood of the professionals and other groups who work within the hospital sector. 'The related slowness of planners, profesionals, voluntary bodies and service-users and their families to agree on a common approach to community care for people with mental health problems has also proved a significant obstacle to progress' (Beardshaw and Morgan, 1990). The policies and attitudes of the past continue to have a major influence on the different roles of relevant agencies and professionals and how they interact.

It is for this reason that this chapter will include details of legislative and practice changes over the last sixty years. An understanding of these changes is crucial when exploring the reasons for poor collaboration particularly between hospital and community services.

Historical background and the role of legislation

Until very recently, legislation has focused on hospital provision and procedures for hospital admission. There has been little legislation which has fostered or encouraged interprofessional collaboration, the building-up of community services or facilities for meeting non-medical need. The reason for this legislative emphasis is partially historical. The large mental asylums were first provided in response to pressure from reformers wishing to improve conditions for the mentally ill. All of those admitted had to undergo compulsory certification. It is perhaps this legacy that has meant that the various laws passed in this century have focused on hospital care and compulsory admission. The Mental Treatment Act passed in 1930 introduced significant changes as it recognised that most patients could be treated voluntarily rather than by compulsion. The Mental Health Act of 1959 provided a number of routes available for hospital admission including informal admission, compulsory admission for observation and compulsory admission for treatment. Patients could be admitted on the grounds of a psychiatric emergency and patients already in hospital could also be detained compulsorily. The Mental Health Act of 1983 also focused on the relevant procedures for compulsory admission. A major objective of the Act was to prevent the abuse of human rights by limiting the administration of treatments to patients without their consent.

These laws have focused on the hospital setting rather than community provision. They have also focused on medical treatment. This is linked to the status of medicine and psychiatry in comparison with other professionals and workers. After the two World Wars, the stature of psychiatry was increased by the success of some of the treatments used during these periods and by 1945 there was a widespread acceptance that the psychiatrist was the expert in mental illness (Butler, 1993). The range of new psychotropic drug treatments developed in the late 1940s and the 1950s reinforced this view. The discovery of antibiotics which brought about a dramatic cut in deaths from infectious diseases led people optimistically to hope that individuals diagnosed with schizophrenia could be 'cured' by drugs such as chlorpromazine. All these developments elevated the position of psychiatry as a profession within medicine and in relation to other groups of workers and professionals.

The National Assistance Act implemented in 1948 gave local authority powers to provide services for the needy. However, what services were provided for the mentally ill remained at the discretion of each local authority and local policies and resources determined the services available (Butler, 1993). The local authorities had to satisfy the needs of their population and facilities for the mentally ill were usually awarded low priority in comparison with the need for housing and better standards of education. While there was an increase in interest in the value of day care for the mentally ill, local authorities did not have the duty to provide it. There were also few staff employed by local authorities who could assist in the rehabilitation of patients from hospitals. Psychiatric social workers were few in number and the only service that local authorities had to provide was the authorised officer needed to make applications for compulsory admissions to hospital.

In 1959 there were no provisions made in the new Mental Health Act to develop integrated services in the community or to encourage further interprofessional collaboration. This omission occured even though there was a growing recognition that community care was more appropriate in many cases than hospital care. The 1962 Hospital Plan was based on statistical projections that indicated a sharply falling need for mental hospital beds. This was linked with the conviction that the large asylums were no longer an appropriate place to provide care (Powell, 1961).

In the 1950s and 1960s, the new policies and treatments led the way to major changes. Patients could be treated quickly and discharged quickly. The revolving door policy posed problems for the management of patients whose illness was episodic in character, especially when the principal device available to professionals was the inpatient service of the hospital with no corresponding facility in the community. Alongside these developments should have been an ongoing resourcing of community services, such as housing, day care and social support, as early discharge meant that patients had needs for other sorts of services in addition to medical care. However, during this period, the number of mental health professionals in the community was relatively small and services were underdeveloped.

One of the alternatives to the old-style asylum which developed in the early 1960s was the appearance of departments of psychiatry within local district general hospitals. This was beneficial in that it encouraged the integration of psychiatry into other parts of the

NHS. Patients were also seen and cared for in their own locality. However, it did not necessarily encourage the development of services outside the hospital or cater for the non-medical needs of patients by developing collaborative links with agencies based outside the hospital.

In 1966 the Ministry of Health was replaced by The Department of Health and Social Security. This body brought together the three strands of health, social services and social security into a single department. As there were still major concerns regarding quality of care, a review of mental health policy was undertaken which resulted in the White Paper 'Better Services for the Mentally Ill' (DHSS, 1975).

The White Paper emphasised the need to develop local community care services. It also indicated that there should be a shift in balance from hospital to community-based care, including the expansion of social services care, day care and social work support. Psychiatric services were encouraged to develop in the district general hospitals but the White Paper recognised that some of the older mental hospitals would continue to have a role in the longer term. It stressed the need for co-ordination between social services, primary health care and the secondary services, and also indicated that increased staffing levels would be necessary to enable individual patient care to be assessed on a multidisciplinary basis. This was important to avoid a deterioration in care for those discharged from hospital to community.

The White Paper was written to give the general direction of long-term policy rather than to suggest immediate changes. It did not give any indication of the resource implications of the new arrangements either in terms of buildings or in staff training and development. New funds were not earmarked for the development of social services for the mentally ill. In fact, the opposite occurred in the social services, with mental health services receiving much less emphasis than before. The 1968 Seebohm Report led to the creation of the social service departments in 1970, and the generic social worker. Although these departments brought about change and development, scarce resources were mostly spent on child care services and in residential provision for the elderly. Social workers previously specialising in mental health, taking on generic roles, often found that child protection was their top priority.

Similarly to the Mental Health Acts before it, the 1983 Mental Health Act did not consider the role of all other forms of intervention such as outpatient and day care or community support. It did not consider the needs of the huge majority of mental health service-users who are not subjected to compulsory treatment (OHE, 1989; Butler, 1993).

The need for change in this direction was recognised by the Audit Commission in their report 'Making a Reality of Community Care' (Audit Commission, 1986). This report indicated that the reduction of NHS hospital provision had been greater than corresponding increases in community services. It produced evidence to show that less than one-third of the planned day centres and less than half the required day hospitals had been created. The report was also critical of the relationships between the health authorities and social services departments. It showed major geographical variations in standards of care developed and inadequate staffing levels. The report stressed the need for bridging finance to develop community provision before reducing hospital services.

Thus the emphasis of the NHS seemed to be on the closure of old hospitals or reductions in the number of hospital beds, rather than an increase in provision of care for individuals in the community. The Commission identifed a number of authorities that had made good progress. Key features of success included service integration focusing on local neighbourhoods, a multidisciplinary approach to working, and partnerships being developed between statutory and voluntary agencies. The recommendations of this report in 1986 were to some extent a prelude to the 1988 Griffiths Report. This in turn prepared the way for the three major white papers of the late 1980s, *Promoting Better Health* (Department of Health, 1987), *Working for Patients* (Department of Health, 1989a) and *Caring for People* (Department of Health, 1989b).

The shift towards community services

In 1987, Sir Roy Griffiths began his review of community care services and produced his report *Community Care: Agenda for Action* in 1988. The Griffiths Review considered that there should be a greater involvement by local government and that resources should be made available for this. He considered that packages of care should be delivered to each individual in need. While the provider of component services could be one of a number of agencies, mechanisms should be in place to deliver comprehensive and integrated services. The Griffiths solution was to name social services departments as the lead agencies to manage and co-ordinate care in the community. In terms of mental health, the emphasis on assessment is specifically limited to those who are thought to require short-term admission to hospital.

The White Paper *Caring for People* was published in November 1989. The central recommendation of the Griffiths Report that social service departments should become the lead agencies in community care provision was accepted. These departments were given authority to hold the budget for residential care, including supporting clients in their own homes. This paper emphasised that for the majority of people community care was preferable to hospital or residential care. This would mean that there would have to be new forms of support for carers and the local authorities would be required to introduce formal assessment procedures and establish case management to reduce the fragmented provision of services. To achieve all of these changes it was essential that a new collaborative arrangement had to be created between health and social care services.

Monies from a variety of sources, including income support and housing benefit would be brought under a single budget managed by the local authorities and this was supposed to be used to fund all aspects of social care for local residents. Social care would include domiciliary, day care and respite services. For those with mental health problems, local authority social services department were to become responsible for the assessment of social need and the development of individual care packages to meet these needs. Local authorities were to set up separate inspectorates to monitor residential care. The health authorities would still be responsible for the assessment of health needs.

Central to the provision of services in *Caring for People* is the system of case management. The proposed core roles of the case manager include the identification of people in need; the delivery of care; monitoring of the quality of care; and reviewing client needs. The case manager acts as purchaser and will be able to draw upon the mixed economy of care in which private and voluntary service providers compete with the statutory sector. At the present time, a major research project is under way into case management (sometimes called care management) for the mentally ill (Clifford and Craig, 1988; Ryan *et al.*, 1991).

Although systems developed vary considerably between authorities (Clifford and Craig, 1988), some care managers may have a mainly managerial role with little direct client contact. In the White Paper, it is clear that it is not essential that the case manager actually carries out all of these tasks personally. This may have the effect of diminishing front-line services and demoralising direct care staff. Care management is also only brought into play where an individual's needs are complex or significant levels of resources are involved.

Many practitioners coming from the health arena are concerned about the likely consequences of the new proceedings (Holloway, 1990). This is especially so with regard to the experience of local authorities in assessing and meeting the social needs of certain groups of individuals such as those identified with 'challenging behaviour'. There are also concerns over the split between social and medical care. The NHS will be expected to provide residential health care while the social services will be a purchaser of residential social care. This is likely to lead to conflict over which agency is responsible for what. Movement of long-stay patients out of hospital into community settings is to result in a transfer of resources from health to social services.

From 1991, a specific care grant was made available. A central fund administered by the Regional Health Authorities has and will provide grants for the development of social care for the mentally ill on the basis of joint plans between health and local authorities. A prime condition for the grant is that it has to be targeted at patients or clients already involved with a specialist psychiatric service. This initiative is intended to act as an incentive for practical joint planning. If co-operation is not possible, the money will not be available. However, the level of this funding is very small (in the first year, £21 million in total from central government, which had to be topped up by the local authorities by £7 million). As this had to be divided between 100 or more social services departments, it does not provide a considerable incentive for joint ventures (Butler, 1993).

Following the publication of *Caring for People*, the Department of Health published circular HC(90)23 which set out ideas on the 'Care Programme Approach' for the mentally ill (Department of Health, 1990). This approach was intended for mentally ill people who are in touch with specialist psychiatric services. In place of the case manager the government guidelines identified the key worker. This person was to keep in touch with the patient and monitor that the agreed health and social care is given. Procedures for those being discharged from hospital will have to be agreed with the local authority and involve a 'care programme' approach in which needs for health and social care are assessed prior to discharge and a named individual is made responsible to ensure that these are met. It is envisaged that these needs will be discussed at a multi-agency meeting prior to discharge at which hospital and community agencies would set out their future involvement. However, these meetings might be extremely difficult to undertake in hospitals where turnover is high. It is likely that CPNs and social workers are likely to the designated key workers in many of these cases once a package of care has been agreed.

It is too early to judge the impact these changes will make on interprofessional collaboration. In many areas, poor collaboration between health and social services may continue and changes will need to be monitored carefully.

Underfunding

Although underfunding is implied in the previous section, its significance in the development (or lack of development) of community services cannot be over-emphasised. Mentally-ill people are not perceived by politicians as being a popular client group amongst the electorate. Generally there has been a lack of consistent public demand to bring about major improvements in services except as a short-term response to a specific scandal or crisis. The 'mentally ill' are therefore usually low on the list of priorities of politicians, whether the latter are based in central or local goverment. This has meant that service development has been slow and constantly underfunded with few community facilities in place. This was recognised to a certain extent by the 1975 White Paper *Better services for the Mentally Ill* when they suggested that there was little hope of the 'kind of service we would ideally like even within a 25-year planning horizon' (Department of Health, 1975).

It is the community sector that has suffered most from underfunding. The government Central Statistics Office (CSO) reported in 1990 that 71 per cent of the cost of direct NHS care for the mentally ill was spent on in-patient services. This was spent on a population of 60,000, a small proportion of the 3.7 million people classified as severely 'ill' in the MHF report (1990).

Perhaps the biggest problem which will be encountered with the government's response, *Caring for People*, (Department of Health 1989a) to Sir Roy Griffiths' proposal, *Community Care: Agenda for Action* (Griffiths, 1988) is the initial failure to 'ring-fence' community care funds, thus continuing this underfunding. Under the new system outlined in the White Paper, the government will transfer to local authorities funds that would previously have been spent by the Department of Social Security on income support and housing benefit for people in community care provision. Before the implementation of this proposal, it was cheaper for social services to admit an elderly or disabled persion to a residential home (funded by social security benefits) than provide services to individuals in their own homes, as the latter was funded by social services. This encouraged the placement of individuals in residential care. Sir Roy Griffiths emphasised that money saved on income support and housing benefit should be ring-fenced for community care. This suggestion was not implemented in *Caring for People*, leaving local authorities the power to spend the extra money elsewhere. Local authority social service departments have other pressing concerns, such as implementing the recent new Children Act. In addition, the majority of social services departments are not managing to work within their budgets and services have had to be cut and new plans for services curtailed. As in the past, mentally-distressed clients may have to lose out to other priority groups such as children who have been abused or where child abuse is suspected. While there are a number of voluntary services in the field of mental health, there is still a need for greater resources to fund and support a wide range of provision.

This consistent underfunding has meant that community services have not been built up and that existing services have been constantly overstretched. Different services and different professionals often consider themselves in competition for funds. This has not encouraged multidisciplinary working or workers, planners and managers spending time with other agencies in consultation.

Methods of improving collaboration

Training and education

In teamwork and collaborative work, it is important for each professional to retain certain unique areas of skill and knowledge in order to maintain a clear identity, while sharing the remaining aspects with others. Whatever organisational structures are in place, there will be a need for multidisciplinary training and education for health care professionals at undergraduate or prequalifying levels and at later career stages. Training needs not only to enhance skills and knowledge but also to change the attitudes of each professional. In terms of mental health, it is important that professionals from the secondary care sector receive extra training so that they can work effectively in the community and in general practice. Users, carers and volunteers should be included at all stages. Mixed groups (for example, users and professionals) have often been shown to have brought about a greater shift in attitudes than those containing professional staff only, but these types of groups will need skilful facilitators (Davies, 1989). Multidisciplinary teams need to learn how to share work effectively. Placing a number of individuals from different backgrounds in the same building or base does not mean that they will start to work together, without any extra effort.

Joint planning

Close collaboration between health services, social services, housing, social security, education, transport and the voluntary sector needs joint planning. This means careful manipulation of the joint planning and joint finance mechanisms, as well as the development of co-operative strategies. As Beardshaw and Morgan (1990) comment: 'one of the biggest problems is the separation – financial, administrative and managerial – of health and social services authorities, and the Family Practitioner Service . . .'. *Caring for People* and the new specific care grant were an attempt to stimulate joint planning. Success will depend on the different objectives, priorities, principles and preoccupations of the various sectors. Users, carers, voluntary agencies and community groups should also be directly involved in the planning process.

Some areas have been successful in developing joint planning. Hood and Whitehead described the system developed in Brighton (1990). Planning in this area is a combined effort between health and social services, with named individuals at unit general manager/ assistant director of social services level from each service producing a five-year plan. The planning document produced was published after consultation with voluntary organisations. In addition, each geographical area has a sector executive group and a sector development group. The executive group includes the area manager of social services, senior health manager, senior clinicians and a local nursing development representative. It has management responsibility to implement the plans and make decisions on local resource allocations. The development group includes users, carers, voluntary organisation representatives and operational staff from social services and health. It advises on issues of policy and philosophy and works on specific projects. The authors of the article indicate that 'this planning system has ensured that as many people and views as possible have been represented, ensuring a responsive approach to local needs and helping people to feel they "own" the changes and developments' (Hood and Whitehead, 1990).

Discussions with self-help groups and user organisations can also enable a wider perspective to be taken. Certain groups of clients, for example black people, are more likely to receive inappropriate care. Yamanoto (1984) found that therapy orientated to the culture and needs of the client led to increased client satisfaction and coping. The high utilisation rates of emergency services at general hospitals is another indication that psychiatric services do not meet the needs of many of their clients. A number of practitioners in the mental health field have considered that the setting-up of a single agency which has responsibility for all aspects of mental health services would be a solution to fragmentation (Holloway, 1990; Butler, 1993). If the case management function in relation to the mentally ill were delegated by the local authority to a consortium, the possibility might emerge for a rational, effective and efficient planning of community psychiatric care at a local level. This was one of the four systems of case management identified by Clifford and Craig (1988).

Catchment areas and sectorisation

Using catchment areas is one way of increasing collaboration (Babigian, 1977; Lindholm, 1983; and Tischler *et al.*, 1972). If professionals are responsible for a specific geographical patch, it becomes easier to communicate and get to know the different agencies which also serve that area and the named individuals within them. Professionals know that they are responsible for all clients in that sector and thus breakdowns in continuity of care are less likely.

The effect of sectorisation has also been studied in the psychiatric service. Lindholm in 1983 found that with sectorisation, services were more accessible, and continuity of care increased as well as patient satisfaction with the service. It is unlikely, however, that all services and agencies will operate using the same geographical areas and patch systems. It is important also that the service develops its own list of priorities and mission statement. For example, the service may decide to focus on the severely and chronically distressed individual and develop systems to identify those in the sector with these problems. This may be preferred to a system whereby clients who walk in and refer themselves are given priority. One problem with the catchment service is that it will not be able to offer more specialised services for those with specific types of distress. Referral may be necessary to these services.

Key workers and case management

A key worker is a named individual who is responsible for the client and for making sure that needs are met by collaborating with various agencies on the client's behalf. At the present time, there is little evidence to suggest that clients with key workers receive a more complete and continuous form of care than those clients in the traditional system (Huxley *et al.*, 1990). It is important, however, that key workers do take into account the client's views when making assessments.

Clients involved in a case management approach should receive a thorough assessment and a care plan drawn up using the facilities of the most appropriate agencies and services. This is a feature of the new programmes being developed subsequent to *Caring for People*. The whole care package is the responsibility of the case manager, who will involve the professionals from the private, voluntary and statutory sectors where appropriate. In some situations, the case manager also administers the budget. There have been a number of studies reporting the use of the case management system. It is probably particularly helpful to those clients with long-term problems who need continuity of care (Challis and Davies, 1986). However, there are concerns that creating a layer of purchasing case managers who have little direct contact with clients may reduce the money available to employ staff to provide the care.

Structural considerations

If the different professions and disciplines are placed in one centre or building, it seems likely that co-ordination may be improved. In general, two models have been developed in this country, primary care teams in general practice settings and community mental health centres. Definitions of community mental health centres vary (Huxley *et al.*, 1990).

Community mental health centres

In Great Britain, the number of community mental health centres (CMHCs) has risen markedly in the last decade and estimates indicate that in 1990 there were probably as many as 160 CMHCs nationally. CMHCs were usually set up with the specific brief to deliver a comprehensive community mental health service. However few, if any, CMHCs in this country have inpatient beds, unlike the situation in the United States. But not all CMHCs are fully multidisciplinary. A national survey of CMHCs in 1988 found that more than half are in fact run by health services staff only, with some 26 per cent managed jointly by health authorities and social services departments. Some CMHCs concentrate on preventive services while others focus on rehabilitative services. Most centres permit referral from a variety of sources, including self-referral (Patmore and Weaver, 1991a).

In the 1960s and 1970s, a large number of community mental health centres were set up in the USA in order to provide care when the large mental institutions were closed. Legislation was passed in 1965 to facilitate their establishment supported by Federal funding (Jones, 1988). These centres were to provide a comprehensive inpatient, outpatient and emergency service and originally 2000 were planned. However, many problems were encountered with them, and less than half of this number are in existence now. In general, it was found that more of the resources of these centres (and worker time) were being spent on clients who were not seriously distressed or disabled than on those clients with more major problems. There were also problems with staff roles (especially in relation to the role of the psychiatrist) and with political and medical opposition. Underfunding was also a common difficulty.

As in the USA, CMHCs in Great Britain are often swamped with referrals of clients (including self-referrals) who have relatively minor difficulties. Clients with major mental health difficulties are less likely to demand help from the service and are more likely to drop out of treatment. Outreach is often necessary to involve this client group with chronic difficulties.

CMHCs cannot be assumed to remove the barriers to interagency and interprofessional communication. Staffing a CMHC with a mix of professionals does not ensure that internally co-ordinated services will result. Professional rivalries can abound when staff from different services start working together based in CMHCs. Social workers and CPNs may have very different conditions of work, including size of caseload, pay levels and holiday entitlement. There can be problems regarding professional lines of management. In addition, CMHCs still have to co-ordinate their work with other services including district general hospitals, primary care teams, voluntary agencies and social services departments, to provide a comprehensive service. It is crucial that CMHCs make proper use of the existing primary care service. The two services should function together in tandem. A number of problems arising with interprofessional collaboration have been documented, such as CPNs restricting access of CMHC staff to their clients in one setting, and in others CMHC staff not wishing to take on clients with a psychotic diagnosis. CMHCs also need to take into account the needs of the user: Dowell and Ciarlo (1983) in their study of CMHCs found that 25–40 per cent of their clientele dropped out of treatment. Client drop out may occur for a number of reasons – these can be positive (successful treatment) or negative (inappropriate services or dissatisfaction with the services provided).

Many areas, however, have found that CMHCs have worked well. Teamwork and team integration can develop if enough attention is given to resolving difficulties between staff and their different terms of service. CMHCs are more likely to be successful in situations where there are few existing services. If existing services are relatively well developed, for example strong primary care teams or a crisis intervention service, it is more important that the CMHCs start off with a clear brief on their target population and the roles of staff members (Huxley *et al.*, 1990).

Primary health care teams

As has been mentioned already, the GP is the professional most likely to be contacted by clients with mental distress and, in most cases, it is the GP whom clients will visit for help with problems with their physical ill health. Thus integration of the primary care team and mental health care system is vital.

GPs have an ongoing responsibility to all patients on their list and in this way differ from all other professionals. Patients are rarely turned away or asked to register elsewhere. This encourages continuity of care. However, GPs will vary according to their own priorities and interests, and the service received by the mentally distressed from GPs may vary enormously. As there has been a gradual trend towards larger group practices, with the proportion of practices with five or more partners trebling between 1970 and 1989 (Taylor, 1991), it is possible that most clients have some choice over the GP they see. However, GP training is necessary to place a greater emphasis on mental health work in order to improve the recognition of problems and subsequent decisions about treatment. Studies on this training have shown that improvement does result with GPs becoming more skilled (Gask, 1992).

The trend over recent years has been for general practice to grow by the employment and attachment of a number of different profes-

sionals. The new contract for GPs (Chisholm, 1990) provided opportunities for increased collaboration, as it removed restricons on the
range and number of staff for whom reimbursement may be obtained under the ancillary staff scheme. In addition, many counsellors were employed using health promotion money available from
running stress clinics (although from 1993, restrictions have now
been placed on the use of this money). With the advent of GP
fundholding, GPs can spent their budget by developing services
offered within the practice. A study conducted by the author of this
chapter in SE Thames Region has indicated that developing psychological services within the practice (by the employment of counsel-
lorsáand psychologists) is a priority area for many fundholding
practices.

A recent study conducted by Thomas and Corney suggests that
attachment schemes and the direct employment of mental health
professionals are now widespread (Thomas and Corney, 1992). In this
study, every general practice was contacted in six randomly selected
health districts in England. Half of the 261 practices had a specific link
with a community psyhiatric nurse, 21 per cent with a social worker,
17 per cent with a counsellor, 15 per cent with a clinical psychologist
and 16 per cent with a psychiatrist (see Table 7.1). These links
included employment, attachment and liaison schemes and the mental health professional using the surgery as a base. One survey conducted in England and Wales found that one in five psychiatrists
spent time in a primary care setting (Strathdee and Williams, 1984)
and a study in Scotland found a higher percentage (Pullen and
Yellowlees, 1988). Between 1980 and 1985 the proportion of community psychiatric nurses working in primary care rose from 8 per
cent to 16 per cent (Brooker and Simmons, 1985). Between 1977 and
1986 the proportion of clinical psychologists working with GPs rose
from 14–17 per cent (Broadhurst, 1977; Hall *et al.*, 1986).

Research has identified a number of advantages in basing mental
health professionals at the primary care level, as they are accessible,
and there are fewer barriers for those seeking help and self-referral.
The service is usually non-stigmatising especially in comparison with
community mental health centres or psychiatric hospitals. Psychiatrists working in clinics in the primary care setting have described
how their greater accessibility and less stigmatising environment
have led to the referral of patients who had avoided contact with the
secondary services for many years. Another advantage is the educational benefits to primary care workers of having easier access to the
skills and advice of a mental health specialist. In addition, the mental

Table 7.1

	Employment/ attachment (%)	Liaison/base (%)	No link (%)
Practice nurse (PN)	81.9	1.9	16.2
Health visitor (HV)	64.7	14.9	20.7
District nurse (DN)	56.0	18.7	25.2
Community psychiatric nurse (CPN)	20.7	27.1	52.3
Social worker (SW)	3.4	17.3	79.3
Clinical psychologist	7.5	7.5	85.0
Psychiatrist	4.1	11.3	84.6
Counsellor	9.4	7.5	83.1

health worker will be able to learn from practice staff and will benefit byáhaving access to background information on clients referred, and this has an interprofessional educational benefit (Strathdee and Williams, 1984; Strathdee *et al.*, 1990).

Their survey identified three working patterns that had emerged for psychiatrists working in primary care; the 'consultation' pattern, the 'shifted outpatient clinic' pattern and the 'liaison-attachment' pattern. 28 per cent of the psychiatrists adopted the 'consultation' pattern in which the specialist held seminars and/or assessed the client but treatment was still administered by the GP. Most (64 per cent) were involved in treatment as well as assessment, either operating a system similar to an outpatient clinic, 'shifted outpatient', or in collaboration with other mental health professionals, the 'liaison-attachment' pattern. Interestingly, the latter pattern was more common in the long-standing schemes where working links between professionals were well-developed.

In addition, there is some evidence that the ethos developed in primary care (that is, long-term responsibility for patients) is reflected in and shared by the professionals attached or employed in this setting. Studies investigating social work attachments to general practice and comparing them with social workers in local authority departments, suggest that those attached to general practice not only were found to make many more contacts with other agencies than the local authority-based social workers, but were more likely to maintain contact with the client when other agencies were involved rather than relinquish it. They worked very much as key workers assuming a longer-term responsibility for each patient much in the same way as the GPs did. Social workers normally conducted a thorough assessment for each client referred by the GP rather than just dealing with the presenting problem. It seemed that the close collaboration between GP and attached social worker and the discussions of work carried out made each side more accountable for their actions. A study of clients' views in the two settings indicated that this was indeed the case, and that clients seen in the health service setting were generally more satisfied with the care received and considered that more of their needs were met (Corney, 1983).

There is, however, one reason to argue that not all community mental health services should be based in primary care settings, particularly in deprived urban areas. Thomas and Corney's study found that there was a tendency for some practices to have many links while others had few. Some practices were more attractive to mental health professionals due to reasons of size, location, facilities or staff. The question arises whether it is the most effective use of resources for some practices to have links with a counsellor, psychologist and CPN while other similarly sized practices have none of these. The patients on the lists of highly collaborative practices may receive a better service (or a better range of services) only at the expense of patients at other less accessible or less amenable practices. This poses questions over equity. If resources are placed into developing multidisciplinary teams based in primary care, patients registered with GPs who do not wish to collaborate will be penalised.

The above is particularly important when services in inner cities are considered. Many GPs who work in inner cities operate either as single-handed practitioners or from poor quality accommodation and are therefore less likely to be able to employ mental health staff or have these attached to the practice. Many studies have shown that chronically distressed clients are more likely to drift to the cities, and it is precisely those areas of multiple deprivation where primary care teams are less likely to be developed.

As with community mental health centres, there often appears to have been an assumption that 'attachment' and similar arrangements were synonymous with the concept of 'teamwork'. Many mental health workers simply 'shift' their clinic from the hospital to the surgery or centre with little or no increase in joint working (Brown *et al.*, 1988). Gilmore and colleagues (1974) studied three primary health care teams. They found that teams do not evolve from attachments without conscious planning based on the promotion of awareness among all team members of what is involved in teamwork and of the factors which hinder and accelerate the process. There are also problems regarding organisational features in general practice: teamwork can be particularly difficult when one member is the employer and another is the employee. As has been previously mentioned, attached staff may also find that they have divided loyalties and commitments.

It is also important to consider, in this context, the small part of the population who are not registered with a GP, and who are homeless (approximately 2 per cent). Schemes are necessary to target this group of individuals. Many of those unregistered are the homeless and a high proportion of these have been found to be chronically distressed. A range of drop-in centres, night shelters and outreach services needs to be developed for this needy group. A study of users of night shelters estimated that over a third of this population was suffering from a mental 'disorder' and this may reflect the consequences of discharging patients from hospital without adequate follow up (Weller *et al.*, 1987).

Conclusions

It is too early to judge whether the reforms proposed in *Caring for People* will bring about major changes in interprofessional collaboration. The changes in general practice (for example GP fundholding), however, are very likely to increase the numbers of mental health professionals working in this setting. In all settings, however, shared training and education is necessary to ensure that collaboration and teamwork occur. In the light of inadequate information on effectiveness, it would seem sensible to pursue several models of community teams simultaneously, with continual reference to the criteria for good practice. There should be properly funded emergency clinics or crisis teams, out-of-hours social work teams, respite care beds and special family therapy in addition to less formal support (Groves, 1990). A mixture of provision should be provided, including day hospitals, day centres, community mental health centres, and primary care teams, as well as centres run by voluntary agencies.

The conventional model of having professionals based in district hospitals appears to have many flaws, except for the highly specialised forms of investigation and treatment. The general practice model and the community mental health centre have a part to play, depending on local needs and initiatives. It has been strongly argued in this chapter that specialist professionals trained in psychiatry should work closely with, or attached to, primary health care teams. This is an option which will guarantee more thoroughly a seamless service which is flexible and provides sustained care in the community for this vulnerable group.

References

Audit Commission (1986), *Making a reality of community care* London: HMSO).

Babigian, H. (1977), 'The impact of CMHCs on the utilization of services', *Archives of General Psychiatry*, 34 (4), pp. 385–94.

Beardshaw, V. and Morgan, E. (1990), *Community Care Works* (London: MIND).

Brewin, C. R., Wing, J. K., Mangen, S. P., Brugha, T. S., MacCarthy, B. and Lesage, A. (1988), 'Needs for care among the long-term mentally ill: a report from the Camberwell High Contact Survey', *Psychological Medicine*, 18, pp. 457–68.

Broadhurst A. (1977), 'What part does general practice play in community clinical psychology?' *Bull. Br. Psychol. Soc.* 30, pp. 304–9.

Brooker, C. and Simmons, S. (1985), 'A study to compare two models of community psychiatric nursing care delivery', *J. Adv. Nursing*, 10 pp. 217–23.

Brown, R., Strathdee, G., Christie-Brown, J. and Robinson, P. (1988), 'A Comparison of Referrals to Primary Care and Hospital Outpatient Clinics', *British Journal of Psychiatry*, 153, 168–73.

Bruce, N. (1980), Teamwork for Preventive Care (Chichester: Wiley).

Brugha, T.S., Wing, J.K., Brewin, C.R., MacCarthy, B., Mangen, S. and Lesage, A. (1988), 'The Problem of People in Long-Term Psychiatric Day Care', *Psychological Medicine*, 18, pp. 443–56.

Butler, T. (1993), *Changing mental health services* (London: Chapman & Hall).

Challis, D. and Davies, B. (1986), *Case management in community care* (Aldershot: Gower).

Chisholm J. W. (1990), 'The 1990 contract: its history and its content', *British Medical Journal*, 300, pp. 853–6.

Clare, A. and Corney, R. (1982), *Social work and primary health care* (London: Academic Press).

Clifford, P. and Craig, T. (1988), *Case management systems for the long term mentally ill* (London: Research and Development for Psychiatry).

Cooper, B. Harwin, B., Depla, G. and Shepherd, M. (1975), 'Mental health in the community, an evaluative study', *Psychological Medicine*, 5, pp. 372–80.

Corney, R. (1980), 'A comparative study of referrals to a local authority intake team with a general practice attachment scheme and the resulting social workers' interventions', *Social Science & Medicine*, 14, pp. 675–82.

Corney, R. (1983), 'The views of clients new to a general practice attachment scheme and to a local authority social work intake team', *Social Science & Medicine*, 17, 20, pp. 1549–58.

Corney, R. (1984), *The effectiveness of social work in the management of depressed women in general practice* (Psychological Medicine Monograph, Cambridge: Cambridge University Press).

Corney, R. (1990), 'A survey of professional help sought by patients for psychosocial problems', *British Journal of General Practice*, 40, pp. 365–8.

Davies, M. (1989), *Doctors, carers and general practice* (London: MSD Foundation, Tavistock House).

DHSS (1975), *Better services for the Mentally Ill*, Cmnd 6233 (HMSO: London).

Department of Health (1987), *Promoting Better Health* (London: HMSO).

Department of Health (1989a), *Caring for People* (London: HMSO).

Department of Health (1989b), *Working for patients* (London: HMSO).

Department of Health (1990), *The Care Programme Approach for people with a mental illness referred to specialist psychiatric services*, HC(90)23, (London: HMSO).

Dingwall, R. (1982), 'Problems of teamwork in Primary Care', in Clare, A. and Corney, R. *Social work and primary health care* (London: Academic Press).

Dowell, D. and Ciarlo, J. (1983), 'Overview of the CMHC', *Community Mental Health Journal*, 19, pp. 95–125.

Gask, L. (1992), 'Training general practitioners to detect and manage emotional disorders', *International Review of Psychiatry*, 4, pp. 293–300.

Gilmore, M., Bruce, N. and Hunt, M. (1974), 'The work of the nursing team in general practice' (London: Council for the Education and Training of Health Visitors).

Goldberg, D. and Blackwell, B. (1970), 'Psychiatric illness in general practice', *British Medical Journal*, 2, pp. 439–43.

Goldberg, D. and Huxley, P. (1980), *Mental illness in the community, the pathway to psychiatric care* (London: Tavistock).

Griffiths, R. (1988), *Community Care: Agenda for action, a report to the Secretary of State for Social Services* (London: HMSO).

Groves, T. (1990), 'What does community care mean now?', *British Medical Journal*, 300, pp. 1060–62.

Gudeman, J. and Shore, M. (1984), 'Beyond deinstitutionalisation', *New England Journal of Medicine*, 311, pp. 832–6.

Hall, J., Koch, H., Pilling, S., Winter, K. (1986), 'Health services information and clinical psychology', *Bull. Br. Psychol. Soc.*, 39 pp. 126–30.

Holden, J. M., Sagovsky, R. and Cox, J. L. (1989), 'Counselling in a general practice setting: controlled study of health visitor intervention in treatment of postnatal depression', *British Medical Journal*, 298, pp. 223–6.

Holloway, F. (1990), 'Caring for people: a critical review of British Government policy for the community care of the mentally ill', *Psychiatric Bulletin*, 14, pp. 641–5.

Holloway, F. (1991), 'Day Care in an Inner City I and II', *British Journal of Psychiatry*, 158, pp. 805–16.

Hood, S. and Whitehead, T. (1990), 'One path to a comprehensive district psychiatric services', *Health Services Management*, August, pp. 174–7.

Hoult, J. (1986), 'Community care of the acutely mentally ill', *British Journal of Psychiatry*, 149, pp. 137–44.

Hunt, M. (1974), 'An analysis of factors influencing teamwork in general medical practice', M.Phil Thesis, Faculty of Social Sciences, University of Edinburgh.

Huntington, J. (1981), *Social work and general medical practice* (London: George Allen & Unwin).

Huxley, P., Hagan, T., Henelly, R. and Hunt, J. (1990), *Effective community mental health services* (Aldershot: Avebury).

Jones, K. (1988), *The experience in mental health-community care and social policy* (London: Sage).

Jones, R. (1992), 'Teamwork in primary care: how much do we know about it?', *Journal of Interprofessiona Care*, 6, pp. 24–9.

Johnstone, E., Owens, D., Gold, A., Crow, T., MacMilln, T. (1984), '*Schizophrenia Patients Discharged from Hospital*' British Journal of Psychiatry, 145, pp. 586–90.

Langsley, D. (1975), 'Community mental health: a review of the literature', in W. Barton and C., Sanborn *An assessment of the CMHC movement* (Lexington, Mass:).

Leff, J. (1993), 'The TAPS Project: Evaluating Community Placement of Long Stay Psychiatric Patients', *The British Journal of Psychiatry*, Vol. 162, supplement 19.

Lee, S. and Murray, R. 'The long-term outcome of Maudsley depressives', *British Journal of Psychiatry*, 153, pp. 741–51.

Lindholm, H. (1983), 'Sectorized psychiatry', *Acta Psychiat. Scand.*, (suppl 304), 67, pp. 1–127.

Mental Health Foundation (1990), *Mental illness: the fundamental facts* (London: MHF).

Office of Health Economics (1989), *Mental health in the 1990s* (London: OHE).

Pantellis, C., Taylor, J., Campbell, P. (1988), 'The South Camden Schizophrenia Survey', *Bull. R. Coll. Psychiatrists*, 12, pp. 98–101.

Parsloe, P. and Stevenson, O. (1980), *Social Services Teams: the Practitioners' view* (London: HMSO).

Patmore, C. and Weaver, T. (1991a), 'Community mental health teams: lessons for planners and managers', *Good Practices in Mental Health*, London.

Paykel, E. S., Mangen, S. P., Griffith, J. H. and Burns, T.P. (1982), 'Community psychiatric nursing for neurotic patients: a controlled study', *Br. J. Psychiatry*, 140, pp. 573–81.

Powell, E. (1961), Speech by the Minister of Health, Report of the Annual Conference of the National Association of Mental Health, London.

Pullen, I. and Yellowlees, 'A. (1988), Scottish psychiatrists in primary health care settings: a silent majority', *Br. J. Psychiatry*, 153 pp. 663–6.

Regier, D., Burke, J., Manderscheid, R. and Burns, B. (1985), 'The chronically mentally ill in primary care', *Psychological Medicine*, 15, pp. 265–73.

Robson, M. H., France, R. and Bland, M., (1984), 'Clinical psychologist in primary care: controlled clinical and economic evaluation', *British Medical Journal*, 288, pp. 1805–8.

Ross, M. and Scott, M. (1985), 'An evaluation of the effectiveness of individual and group cognitive therapy in the treatment of depressed patients in an inner city health centre', *Journal of the Royal College of General Practitioners*, 35, pp. 239–80.

Ryan, P., Ford, R. and Clifford, P. (1991), 'Case management and community care', *Research and Development for Psychiatry*, London.

Sayce, L. (1987), *CMHCs Conference Report, National Unit for Psychiatric Research and Development*, London.

Scott, A. and Freeman, C. (1992), 'Edinburgh primary care depression study: treatment outcome, patient satisfaction and cost after 16 weeks', *British Medical Journal*. 304, pp. 883–7.

Shepherd, M., Cooper, B., Brown, A. and Kalton, G. (1966), *Psychiatric illness in general practice*, (Oxford: Oxford University Press).

Skuse, D. and Williams, P. (1984), 'Screening for psychiatric disorders in general practice', *Psychological Medicine*, 14, pp. 365–77.

Strathdee, G., Brown, R. and Doig, R. (1990), 'A standardised assessment of patients referred to primary care and hospital psychiatric clinics', *Psychological Medicine*, 20, pp. 219–24.

Strathdee, G. and Williams, P. (1984), 'A survey of psychiatrists in primary care: the silent growth of a new service,' *J.R. Coll. Gen. Prac.* 34 pp. 615–18.

Taylor D. (1991), *Developing Primary Care* (London: King's Fund Institute Research Report 10).

Teasdale, J. D., Fennell, M. J. V., Hibbert, G. A. (1984), 'Cognitive therapy for major depressive disorder in primary care', *British Journal of Psychiatry*, 144, pp. 400–6.

Tischler, G., Henisz, J., Myers, J. and Garrison, V. (1972), 'Catchmenting and the use of mental health services', *Archives of General Psychiatry*, 27, pp. 389–92.

Thomas, R. and Corney, R. (1992), 'A survey of links between mental health professionals and general practice in six district health authorities', *British Journal of General Practice*, 42, pp. 358–61.

Thomas, R. and Corney, R. (1993), 'General practitioners' attitudes to mental health professionals: a survey, *British Journal of General Practice*. *British Journal of Psychiatry*, 145, pp. 9–14.

Weller, B., Weller, M., Coker, E., Mahomed, S (1987), 'Crisis at Christmas, 1986' *Lancet*, 553–4.

World Health Organisation (1973), *Psychiatry and primary medical care* (Copenhagen: WHO Regional Office for Europe).

Yamanoto, J. (1984), 'Orienting therapists and patients needs to increase patient satisfaction', *American Journal of Psychiatry in Medicine*, 9, pp. 339–50.

8 *Palliative care*

Patricia Owens

Chapter summary

This chapter addresses the issues of death and the care of those with serious chronic or terminal illness. The power of professional groups such as doctors is discussed in relation to the development of technology, the prolongation of treatments and the social and financial costs. The author sets current practices within the context of cultural imperatives, and draws upon historical and anthropological material to illustrate the increasing isolation of individuals dying within our health and social care systems. The importance of an interdisciplinary approach is explored, and the improvement of training for all professionals at both pre-clinical and post-qualifying levels.

The role of medicine and the management of death

Major changes in demographic and epidemiological trends have affected the nature of our services. Death caused by communicable diseases such as cholera, TB, smallpox, syphilis and typhoid in our society in the nineteenth century have been overcome by external and internal interventions. Public health measures and the introduction of effective treatments and improved nutrition have in turn affected the role of medicine and the pattern of ill health in the community (McKeown, 1979 Lewis, 1986).

The concept of the body as a machine which can be improved by surgical and medical intervention has become part of our everyday understanding of health care. However, Illich (1977) has severely criticised this view as one that positively contributed to the generation of ill health, and reduces the capacity of individuals to care for themselves, endure suffering and face death. New drugs or medical and surgical interventions have given the medical profession the power to prolong life even in the face of outcomes such as severe long-term disability and physical and mental suffering. Illich contends that medicine has become 'a defence against death', as death outside old age is perceived as unnatural and preventable. Blame is to be attached if it occurs, as doctors and nurses are believed to have failed. Natural death, unless it occurs in old age, has almost become a civil right for citizens of developed countries.

These ideas are controversial, and have strong philosophical overtones in terms of how we perceive illness, and the ethical and legal responsibilities of doctors and other professionals involved in health and community care. Kennedy (1981) challenged the increasing power of the medical profession in *The Unmasking of Medicine*. Huge advances in medical technology had put the medical profession in a position of unprecedented power, but the capacity to prolong life is coupled with the generation of new and complex moral dilemmas. When, where and how a person dies may become a situation which is largely determined by the expertise of the doctor.

This power over life and death was recently illustrated by the case of Dr Cox (*The Times*, 1992 and 1993) who, responding to repeated requests from a patient to end her life, took an active step, and did so by prescribing a lethal drug. This action was not accepted as ethical or lawful by a nursing member of the health care team. The case raised a public debate about the patient's role in decision-making in the face of long-term degenerative illness and death, and the responses of the doctor. The court, while finding the doctor guilty, accepted that there were mitigating circumstances in terms of the patient's attitude and extreme physical and long-term suffering. Dr Cox was given a suspended sentence for attempted murder. However, this case serves to illustrate the courts' own preference to use a scientific model to define the proper conduct of a doctor.

What is significant about this case is that the doctor and nurse did not have a shared view of how to approach the suffering of the patient, Mrs Lilian Boyer, and control her pain. The death of this patient in these circumstances to some extent is an illustration of the absence of an interprofessional approach. Kennedy (1981) has identified the development of the singular and almost magical power and autonomy of the doctor as a feature of modern medical practice. This encourages the doctor to assume an authority over other professionals and the patients. However, he comments that medical education makes the doctor poorly adjusted for the reality of the working world.

In addition to this mythologisation of medicine, and the concept of the physician as powerful healer and scientist, there is the idea derived from Hippocratic principles that if the doctor has the freedom to treat and care, the patient has similar freedoms to receive such care and treatments. Linked to these options is the idea of choice, and a growing emphasis on the rights and entitlements of the patient with respect to access to health. These primary elements underlie, in part, the developing market philosophy in health care and its accompanying effects outlined in earlier chapters.

From the doctor's point of view, choosing to continue to treat a condition that is terminal may involve making decisions concerning the relative costs of drugs and the quality of a life prolonged by such treatments (Calabresi and Bobbitt 1978). This presents society with a dilemma as there are tensions between the growing power of the professionals in determining those choices, the economic and bureaucratic restraints on that power, and the freedom of the patient to choose to pursue remission or terminate treatments, and face death sooner rather than later. There are no comfortable formulae to facilitate this process. But it seems that we are moving more and more towards a fiercely competitive business environment in which power is centralised into the hands of an elite of technocrats, who control the activities of doctors by rationing resources.

In the health care system in the USA the idea that death can be avoided indefinitely is a position reinforced by the legal system and an adversarial climate, in which litigation surrounds the question of the withholding of treatments. Access to medical records, and the patient's right to know has led to the development of the doctrine of 'informed consent', and this has meant that patients now participate more fully than before in decisions about prolonging life or accepting that a fatal disease takes its natural course. But freedom in this context is somewhat illusory, as market forces may determine that one person's freedom is at the expense of another's. The question arises whether freedom to choose as a right is more important than equal access to health care resources.

Illich's assertion that medical science has been ascribed almost magic power, and has come to be seen as a defence against death, means that health care teams are faced with situations, expectations and choices that hitherto did not exist. It is debatable in these circumstances, whether in the future the lone doctor can make or be expected to face these decisions entirely alone. Consequently, health care professionals need to be educated together to find new ways of working to provide not only a unified approach to the dying person in order to prevent over- treatment, but also to find strategies for developing support systems which maximise the quality of a patient's life an death, and ensure that professionals, patients and their carers are involved in the making of decisions about palliative and terminal stages of care.

It is important at this stage to emphasise the need for the doctor to be seen as part of a team, alongside other professionals caring for patients. Increasingly the doctor is in the unenviable position of being not only the patient's *advocate* but is also a *servant of the state*. In these circumstances, a mutual support structure is necessary for professionals, so that any decision is made with reference to a clear code of conduct shared by all those working in the team, and understood and accepted by the patient.

The case of Graham Pink, the charge nurse who criticised staffing levels on a ward for elderly people with acute illnesses, also illustrates this point. The nurse in this instance found it impossible to provide what he deemed a reasonable standard and quality of care for the patients on his ward. Charge Nurse Pink was distressed by the frequent situations which occurred where patients were dying alone and untended in distressing circumstances. He was isolated in his fight for better staffing levels, and was portrayed by the press and by his managers as having little or no support from his colleagues. He finally lost his job, but through a sustained campaign, has won the right at Department of Health level for individual 'whistleblowers' to be heard in the NHS (Brindle, 1990a, b).

This case demonstrates the problem of the role conflict that can occur when management of resources, professional duty to the employer and ethical considerations in terms of patient care, have to be weighed up and difficult but acceptable choices made. It is not within the power of an individual professional, be he or she a doctor or a nurse, to find answers to these complex questions alone.

Cultural attitudes to death

But have technological, legal and social transformations created the depersonalisation of death and its processes in our society? Gorer (1965), a social anthropologist writing about his own searing experience of losing a much-loved brother, described the anguish he suffered because he was unable to mourn publicly or express his grief. Gorer's personal experience and subsequent conclusion was that death is the final taboo in advanced industrial societies. Almost twenty years on, Kellehear (1984) expressed it in another way, suggesting that we have developed 'a death-denying culture'. These cultural attitudes create a difficult and complex working environment for the health care professionals, who have to face and evaluate their own personal attitudes and actions as well as those of their clients and patients, and society itself.

Ariès in *The Hour of Our Death: Western Attitudes to Death* (1981) analysed what he termed rejection of the idea of mortality, observing that in Western society, death and dying have become processes and events which must be 'hushed up'. People no longer die at home, with their family around, but more often in hospital alone, and dying is frequently viewed as a result of failure by doctors to heal. Death is thus defined as a technical phenomenon that happens because care ceases, and is thus related to decisions made by the doctor and the team, and not a natural and unavoidable event (Glaser and Strauss, 1966). An illustration of this was when a doctor, describing modern dilemmas for terminal care in a television documentary on medicine and elderly care in Florida, dryly remarked that in being expected to carry out life-prolonging procedures which did little to improve quality of life for many patients that demanded them, he played along with the idea that 'death is optional'.

All these assertions are based on the belief or knowledge that concepts of death have changed over time in our own society. Western attitudes to death also differ profoundly from those prevalent in other cultures with different belief systems concerning health, illness, death and the afterlife, and existing in vastly dissimilar material circumstances.

Changing attitudes to death on a more general level can be related to the evolution of thought in Western philosophy, which ultimately favours the uniqueness and importance of the individual. The liberty of the individual is the cornerstone of our thought and practice (Gittings, 1984). Evidence of our preoccupation with the individual in the context of attitudes to death is derived from the development of personalised tombs and graves, and other factors such as the growth of the portrait, the novel, the biography and the general iconography associated with death (Stone, 1979). In her study of Western funeral rites, Gittings traces a movement away from community or group responses to death to the modern phenomenon of death being hidden away in hospitals and not openly discussed, but surrounded by fear and embarrassment.

Funeral rites in medieval European societies were prolonged and overt, collective rather than individualistic in approach, emphasising group solidarity and support of the bereaved. They were similar in nature to those described by anthropologists Malinowski (1974), Turner (1969), Van Gennep (1965) and Bloch and Parry (1982) in other cultures. The elaborate and prolonged processes and rituals associated with dying are concerned with reintegration of the dead and the bereaved in the community. The three characteristics of all rituals defined by Van Gennep – those of separation, transition and integration – were integral to providing a recognition of death, affording it meaning in terms of the world-view of a particular society, and giving the living the support from the community to sustain them during the period of bereavement.

Gittings concluded that there is historical evidence that indicates a growing anxiety about death, and the eighteenth-century development of embalming techniques suggests that there was an increasing preoccupation with the preservation of the individual after death. The nineteenth century saw the introduction of mourning clothes which further symbolised the withdrawal of the family of the deceased, and the more central role of kin, to the exclusion of the wider social group. The twentieth-century total abandonment of such formal mourning procedures in our own society is, according to Gittings, a manifestation of the rejection of the reality of death and human grief.

In the face of changes in conceptions about death and the afterlife, and the emergence in Western cultures of the primacy of the individual, professionals are expected to fill the yawning gaps that have occurred in society's support structures. It is difficult to assert that traditional methods of caring for dying people were necessarily more complete or better than in the present, but it does appear that the social isolation of the individual described in so many texts on care of terminally sick people cannot be divorced from more profound shifts in our social responses to death over time.

However, it is easy to romanticise about the past, and to gloss over the terrors of dying, for example, in the workhouse in nineteenth-century England, or the anonymity and disgrace of the pauper's grave. In analysing the significant effects of advances in medical technology and its counterproductive outcomes, it is possible to overlook the more positive developments in the growth and universal accessibility of health care in our society, literally from the cradle to the grave.

Nevertheless, the secularisation of many funeral rites, and the changes and varied nature of spiritual beliefs in our society means that dying presents professionals with human needs that must be met, that exceed the provision of material comfort, treatments and resources. As over 70 per cent of people in England and Wales die in institutions, professionals such as Charge Nurse Graham Pink and Dr Cox are continually faced with the processes of dying which are hidden from the general view. The isolation of the individual in modern society, and the rejection and denial of death directly impact on the professionals working closely with patients in the terminal stages of disease.

When curing stops

The idea that medicine can cure all physical ills has heightened the sense of impotence and failure experienced by health care professionals in the face of those diseases that remain unconquered, as yet, by the advances in scientific treatments. Diseases such as multiple sclerosis, motor neurone disease, Parkinson's disease and Huntington's chorea are responsive to palliative care but not to cure. These diseases that ultimately lead to death are severely disabling over a long period, not only to the sufferers, but to their carers and families. Dying can be a long drawn-out process, and demands of care necessitate complex, sensitive and sustained responses from health and social care professionals working as a team across agency boundaries (Owens, 1987).

Cancer as a condition strikes fear into the hearts of most of us, but more recently with the introduction of new drugs and treatments, this fear has diminished, and it has come out of the closet, and is more openly discussed in the media. The possibility of cure exists with some drug and radiotherapy treatments, and, if not cure, lengthy remission periods. None the less, sufferers and carers still have difficulty in acknowledging the presence of the disease and it remains surrounded by taboos. Doctors lack the training and necessary skills to break bad news about prognosis, and that further interventions are not recommended, or that the condition is in the terminal stages.

More importantly, cancer has been overtaken by the greater and more apocalyptic fear that surrounds AIDS. Kubler-Ross (1987) wrote that hospices in the USA were in a double-bind, in which they feared losing the financial support from cancer patients and their relatives, and for this reason were only allocating 16 per cent of beds to AIDS patients. She movingly described her own experiences in workshops for sufferers in her book *AIDS: The Ultimate Challenge*, and wrote that this disease was the largest socio-political issue in health, dividing religious groups and providing a battleground for medical research. She described the impact on health care teams, 'Many health care professionals themselves treated AIDs patients worse than leprosy patients, often keeping them waiting for hours or until they passed out in a little side room, where they have been placed and forgotten' (1987). Behaviour of staff was described as rejecting and isolating: for example, the strategies of using masks and gowns, and standing about six feet away while interviewing patients emphasised the social and psychological distance that professionals wished to impose between themselves and sufferers.

The profound loneliness and isolation associated with this disease was strongly related to the guilt felt by patients. This guilt in the USA context at first was associated with homosexuality and the marginal status of this group in society. Admission of this fact to families was a major part of the difficulty many patients experienced in gaining support of carers. Men and women who had infected partners or their children also could not rely on that support being available, the whole relationship being distorted by their own guilt in transmitting the disease.

Kubler-Ross frankly described her own sense of repulsion and lack of acceptance, her feeling that this was a disease and a death reserved for other people. At the same time she experienced a sense of horror at the 'final solution' type attitude that prevailed in some quarters. For cancer, she wrote, it seemed there was 'a listening ear', as this was something that could happen to anyone, and rarely was blame attached to individual behaviour. But the connotation of reprehensible sexual behaviour hung over AIDS compounding the sense of shame and guilt experienced by sufferers. The deep feelings of failure that characterised professional responses to incurable diseases in the past were unequivocally expressed in fear and avoidance behaviour in this particular context.

But this is nothing new, only a more extreme and overt expression of societal attitudes to the so-called incurable patient. Sheila Cassidy, in the introduction to 'Final Gifts' (Callanan and Kelley, 1992), wrote 'Because each of us fears death we are tempted to ignore, to marginalise the dying. They are finished, almost finished, while we are busy, at the height of our powers. Their time is over, out time is now; we are on the stage, they are in the wings . . .'. The isolation of the individual carer, be it a relative, friend or professional is also a factor which needs recognition, and strategies developed for counteracting negative effects of rejection of the patient.

The hospice movement and multidisciplinary approaches

Cicely Saunders' pioneering work for cancer sufferers in the hospice movement in this country is based on a philosophy of an interdisciplinary approach which aims to reduce the social and psychological isolation of death in the health care system. Not only does she advocate teamwork, but also a multidimensional concept of care which incorporates emotional and spiritual elements with the practical tasks of pain relief and physical care of dying people (Saunders, 1989, 1993).

A basic principle of the hospice movement is to provide a flexible response to the expressed and perceived needs of patients in the terminal stages of cancer, and to their carers. Mutidisciplinary working is essential in palliative care services in order to respond sensitively to the expressed and perceived needs of patients in the terminal stages of disease. Saunders *et al.* (1990) in the volume *Hospice and Palliative Care: An Interdisciplinary Approach*, give a wide overview of strategies and suggestions for developing successful teamwork for caring for terminally ill patients. These are briefly summarised in the following pages.

Jackson (1990) recommends that team members should be selected on the basis of professional competence, flexible approach, sense of humour, respect for others, ability to support colleagues, and an awareness of what is meant by trust. A multidisciplinary team should have a shared concept of the 'common tasks' and 'accepted objectives'. To achieve these, some professional traditions may need to be adjusted or modified. This makes it possible for individual team members to abdicate roles without loss of face, and creates a stronger group.

It is essential that the team has a recognised leader who takes final responsibility, has purpose and vision, is able to listen with respect, and support individual and collective actions. It is also suggested that other important ingredients of successful teamwork are: developing a shared language among all professionals, having regular meetings together in a comfortable room with minimal interruption, regular meetings with other professionals and agencies, and invitations extended to visit the service and share knowledge (Jackson, 1990).

West (1990) suggests that in interactions with patients it is of central importance not to overwhelm them by having too many professionals around a bed so that the relationship with the patient appears dualistic, and also that the patient should wherever possible, take the leading role. Meetings with the family or primary carers can generate fear, so the agenda should be set in advance and seating arrangements carefully planned, and a professional clearly identified as the leader. Assessment visits should be done only by a professional who has experience of a particular disease, its probable prognosis, and the ability of the carers to provide support at home (Jackson, 1990).

The processes of developing trust in the palliative care team mean not only being able to blur roles, but also to accept that confidentiality means that not everyone has to know everything, and that permission must be sought from the patient to share confidences with others. This is a particularly difficult problem and needs a clear and unambiguous policy. It is by no means certain that everyone has to know everything (Harris, 1990).

Problems that can inhibit successful team work are pressure of work which then disallows time and space for meetings and exchange of ideas, personal problems of team members, poor communication, inadequate resources, management battles and unrealistic expectations of each other. Problems of low staffing can lead to disputes over quality, as in the Graham Pink case, and to individual burn-out. The introduction of new team members is also a potential source of stress and strain, as for a time that person will be viewed as an outsider or intruder which can have a dysfunctional effect.

The central problem for care of cancer sufferers is pain control (Baines, 1990), although weakness and anorexia are also common. To treat patients successfully in this situation it is essential to have regular meetings of the team. In the process of addressing this physical problem, professionals have to also tackle the effects of anger and despair experienced by the patient and staff. The intractability and rapid progression of some cancers and other degenerative conditions such as motor neurone disease also require, in addition to skilled physical care, that professionals should spend time listening and empathizing with the patient and carers. The importance of respite care in these conditions to provide relief for the carers, symptom control for the patient and physical reassessment and readjustments to the environment at home, also needs close cooperation between the primary health care team and the palliative care service (Owens, 1987).

Channon (1990) suggests that all planning of care should involve the patient, and take into account his or her natural preferences for particular team members. The privacy of the patient and those closest to them is of central importance. There should be the careful provision of adequate opportunity to say goodbye to loved ones. Once the patient has died, relatives and carers need the opportunity to rehearse the details of the illness and go over the death, and in so doing be encouraged to accept its reality. The individual preferences of the bereaved should be respected to cry and grieve openly or otherwise, or to sit with the body. These basic principles of the hospice philosophy should enable a team member of any professional group to perform these duties of care (O'Brien, 1990).

The problem of patients with intractable symptoms can be a source of great tension with palliative care teams (Wood 1990). Sometimes there is a mismatch between the expectations of professionals, patients and carers. A balance has to be struck between optimism and pessimism. Team members can feel angry at their failure to alleviate symptoms, and it is essential in these circumstances that the professional group share their feelings of blame and stress. At the same time, patients may use symptoms to gain attention or conversely deny their illness, and the team needs to develop a shared approach to each situation.

Within teams there are sometimes individual professionals who find it difficult to co-operate, particularly in circumstances when the patient, family and professionals have a conflict of views. Often they are defensive about their own professional status, or are people who like to do their own thing, or who want to be everything to everyone. This may be the outward expression of a team member looking to the service to fulfil their own needs rather than those of the patient. They characteristically become over-involved and have a tendency to take no responsibility for the team (Channon, 1990).

The palliative care team have the difficult task to face of accepting that they cannot fix every thing. Lunn (1993) wrote, 'The genius of the hospice interdisciplinary ideal, and the salvation of those of us who work with it is that we do not have to say "I don't know" alone, there is always a combined response.' It is a system, he thinks, that resists professional hierarchy and intellectual snobbery. Palliative care allows for patients, carers and professional to explore feelings and express them rather than formulate answers. Questions of guilt, punishment and forgiveness are explored. 'There is a profound untidiness within the order of the interdisciplinary team', which is associated with each member being available to deep human need and is unrelated to clinical or professional expertise (Lunn, 1993).

Saunders also addresses the need for mutual support in challenging situations, such as when patients say they want to die, or be killed, or allowed to die. These are ethical problems that need open discussion and free expression. But differences in salaries and qualifications lead to inequalities in the power structure within a group and act as barriers which impair communication: for example, when the doctor prescribes and the nurse may administer a drug. This situation, which characterised the Dr Cox case, leads to a failure to take a common approach to the problem of pain relief and a patient's request to die. A non-hierarchical approach within teams is therefore recommended to overcome these problems. Other important facets of palliative care teamwork should be understood and agreed; for example, the question of whether a deceased person still has the right of confidentiality. Do professionals have a right to know and discuss everything about a patient? Should staff avoid collusion with carers and be the patient's advocate before all else? These, and other ethical problems need to be faced jointly by the palliative care team in their own and the patient's interests.

There are significant difficulties in attempting to codify ethical behaviour which need recognition: because of its unrestricted terms of reference, there can be no simple rules. Benjamin and Curtis (1981) suggest that the ethical framework had to be repeatedly applied, tested, refined and revised in the medical and nursing context. The exercise of personal ethical autonomy is constrained by external factors such as the law, the hierarchical nature of most health care teams, and institutional policies.

The interface between the hospital and home

The hospice movement focused primarily on the cancer patient. However, the similarities between the final stages of cancer, AIDS and other degenerative illness are undeniable. The unpleasant symptoms, the enforced dependency, the inability to provide self-care and accompanying psychological changes are common to the end-stage of many chronic illnesses. The home care team is faced with the same tasks already identified in the hospice setting. However, there are differences, as delivering a service can become more intensely personal in the home setting, as the individual nurse or doctor in attendance is frequently alone in coping with the impact of the terminal stages of an illness on the sufferer and the carers (Owens, 1987).

The patient who has been discharged from hospital may have felt reluctant to leave, as there is a fear that all hope is gone and all treatment stopped. The transition from hospital to home has to be co-ordinated, with adequate discharge notice and information, and a planned approach to the patient's care at home (Pritchard *et al.*, 1979). The purpose is to maximise the patient's quality of life right up to the end (Hull *et al.*, 1989). The development of the Terminal Care support team at St Bartholomew's Hospital in London introduced exciting changes in the care of dying people in the acute hospital setting (Dunlop and Hockey, 1990). This innovation created a greater commitment of health care professionals to improve palliative care, and spread this attitude to other ward staff including ward clerks, technicians and secretaries.

The care of dying patients in general hospitals orientated to cure has usually meant that as an aspect of acute service in general it has low priority, and patients have received poor care as a result. The St Bartholomew's support team found that by positively dealing with relatives' and patients' fears about dying, more patients were able to die at home or in the hospice. However, as elsewhere, the majority of patients still continued to die in hospital. The three main reasons why a patient died in hospital were that the patient denied the illness and had made no contingency plans, or carers at home were unable to cope, or the patient was unable to accept transfer elsewhere as the illness progressed. Ward staff caring for these patients generally were found to lack support in the ward situation to deal with distressing symptoms and psychosocial difficulties. Nurses felt ill-equipped professionally, and doctors suffered feelings of helplessness because they were uncertain how to treat some aspects of suffering. Dunlop and Hockey (1990) reported that these factors often led to patients being ignored on ward rounds.

The support team carried out the tasks of advising staff about relief of symptoms, providing counselling and other practical help to patients, generally supporting ward staff, and providing education programmes. There were tensions when consultants believed that the principle objective of the team was merely to transport the patient to the hospice or elsewhere, and empty the bed, even in circumstances when this was not the patient's choice. Similarly, dealing with primary care teams was also problematic, as often GPs and community nurses were unwilling to use powerful opiates to relieve severe pain, and this sometimes led to conflict. Differences in the hospice's philosophy also sometimes meant that there was a reluctance to take a patient if they were still receiving any kind of proactive treatment.

It remains the case that many more people die from cancer in hospital than at home. There are a number of reasons for this, some already touched upon. There is a belief among palliative care teams and patients that only hospital or the hospice can provide adequate pain relief or control of distressing symptoms and there is some evidence to support this view. The patients themselves often believe that as long as they are in hospital there is some hope of a cure. The question health care professionals need to pose is what is in the best interests of the patient? Professionals may feel that a patient is better off in the hospital or hospice, but that person may think and feel differently, and be under the misapprehension that there is little choice (McNulty, 1978). There are no absolute criteria for deciding whether a patient remains at home – each case has to be considered individually (Dunlop and Hockey, 1990)

Emotional problems encountered with carers of dying people can be overwhelming. Professionals will be expected to deal effectively with anger, bitterness, resentment, denial, grief and fear. Their task is to help the patient and carers towards a sense of acceptance. The intensity of this experience in the home situation with no other staff around may lead to burn-out if professional carers are not adequately supported (Owens, 1987). The collapse of home care can lead to a great sense of guilt in the family and among the professionals. The primary health care team has to anticipate the physical, practical and psychological problems that are likely to present themselves, and develop strategies for dealing with them.

McNulty 1978 wrote that the patient may suffer from what is know as a 'conspiracy of silence', particularly in situations where adults are trying to protect children from the reality of death. This may result in the patient being removed to hospital for reasons other than their own good, heightening the sense of alienation and rejection that is experienced in these circumstances. These and other problems of bereavement and unresolved grief can mean that the care team has to continue involvement with a family long after the patient has died.

Implications for the education of health care professionals

What is clear from the literature on palliative care in the home, hospital and hospice is that it is an area which needs special attention in the training of all professional groups. Currently home care teams have developed using specialist workers either from such services as the St Christophers Hospice, the Macmillan and Marie Curie nursing service, or services like the St Bartholomew's Hospital Terminal Care Support Team within the acute hospital structure. The main logic for providing specialist services is that this particular aspect of health care is orientated to responding to patient's complex needs in a holistic way, and that some element of protected time and space is necessary to enable this to happen.

However, it is also evident from an analysis of the literature that much of the training for palliative and terminal care takes place at the post-qualification stage. It seems that doctors, nurses, and other professionals who are in daily contact with people in the final stages of degenerative disease or terminal cancer or AIDs are likely to have had little training at pre-qualification level in dealing with these situations, or a highly developed consciousness of the importance of teamwork. The interdisciplinary approach developed and advocated by Cicely Saunders has been concentrated hitherto on the palliative care of cancer sufferers. The advent of AIDS has created new challenges for terminal care services, but these approaches should be universally applied, as, after all, people are dying all the time of other causes, sometimes slowly and in pain, and it follows that they need the same kind of attention from hospital and primary care teams as those in the hospice.

The cases of Dr Cox and Graham Pink illustrated, among other things, the isolation and despair that can be experienced by professionals in the face of death. The importance of mutual support systems in dealing with terminal care is all too clear from examination of these two dramatic situations. The issues of dying with dignity and limiting suffering for patients and carers rarely can be settled by individual professionals acting independently. This paternalistic attitude of the past needs to be abandoned in the interests of patients, their carers and the professionals themselves.

Kellehear (1984) commented that hitherto medical students have not been prepared for their experiences with death and dying, even though, compared with average non-medical people they are exposed to an 'astronomical amount'. He wrote that medical students have frequently been reported to express fear of death. But in the total care of dying patients it is not just doctors who are involved, and it should, therefore, be considered to be an important part of the curriculum of all professional groups who participate in this process. There is a need not only to cover the technological approach, but to incorporate in training the holistic and multidisciplinary method developed by the hospice movement. This system of care confronts the death-denying culture that has developed in response to the technological cure-all philosophy, by including the spiritual and psychological elements of the dying process as central to palliative care. But in releasing us all from the hushing-up and denial associated with death, new challenges have been created and must be faced by nurses, doctors, social workers and others in the health care system, and these should be approached within the context of a multidisciplinary team offering mutual support.

Members of the palliative care team need to learn how to tell bad news, negotiate or decide when curing stops, estimate quality of life, deal with anguish and suffering which has a psychological as well as a physical dimension, and appreciate the contributions of other professionals to this process. Above all, they need to learn how to deal with and recognise their own attitudes and emotions without guilt or fear. The multidisciplinary approach developed by the hospice movement has provided a model which, ideally, could be included in the curriculum of all health care professionals at the pre-qualification stage of their education. By providing shared learning opportunities for doctors, nurses, social workers and others, professionals will be able to deal more effectively with the reality of their working situation, and develop greater confidence in themselves and others.

The case of Graham Pink has been widely used to illustrate the importance of the individual contribution of 'whistleblowers' and patient advocates in the NHS: that is, the right of professionals to draw attention to low standards of service or deficiencies in care without fear of reprisal by employers. Each professional carries around in his or her head an idea of their ethical framework and their corresponding personal values, and this needs public expression from time to time. An important facet of the sad story of the lonely and undignified deaths of elderly people on Graham Pink's ward is that there was no shared view of the situation. The isolation of elderly patients in the terminal stages of illness in this hospital simply reflected their marginal status in society itself. Charge Nurse Pink drew attention to the facts and to his own professional and personal conflicts, but by acting alone had little success in changing the situation.

Consideration of this case reinforces the view that it is only by developing a shared philosophy of care and agreed policies with members of the health care team which includes doctors, nurses and managers, that these situations can be avoided and standards improved and monitored consistently. Dr Cox, when he returned to work (*The Times*, 3 Februry 1993), was recommended to be attached to a Palliative Care Unit and attend team meetings.

Conclusions

The continued preference for shutting away death in institutions means that professionals are expected to deal expertly and efficiently with it. Relatives will be quick to complain about uncaring professionals, sometimes in an attempt to assuage their own guilt and inability to provide support. But transferring the problem of dying to an institutional setting, may simply be passing it on to professionals who are no better prepared than relatives to provide for all aspects of palliative and terminal care.

The philosophy of the hospice movement has forced professionals to see themselves as part of society, not divorced from it, and as sharing a common humanity with their patients. This has resulted in the removal of barriers that have hitherto protected them from involvement. In these circumstances it is vital that professionals provide each other with support, so that future nurses and doctors do not feel like Graham Pink and Dr Cox that they are individuals alone, left to cope with their own emotions and the complexities and impossible choices of terminal care. Each professional needs to be part of the development of a recognised and shared philosophy of care which supports a total comprehensible system.

Finally, the restrictions on financial resources also mean that professionals are having to find the most efficient and effective ways of delivering care. The flexibility of the team approach helps to avoid duplication of effort and unnecessary treatments, and consequently the patient and carers will receive a more responsive service. But this will only happen if all members have a shared view of the means as well as the ends of a service. On a more abstract level, it has been argued in this chapter that the development of the team approach can be interpreted as a return to the earlier practices of communal sharing of grief and loss. The philosophy of palliative care as expressed by the hospice movement succeeds in incorporating more recent notions of respect for individual rights, along with earlier ideas of group support and community affiliation.

References

Ariès, P. (1981), *The Hour of Our Death: Western Attitudes to Death* (London: Allen Lane).

Baines, M. (1990), 'Tackling Total Pain', in C. M. (ed.), *Hospice and Palliative Care: An interdisciplinary approach* (London: Edward Arnold).

Benjamin, M. and Curtis J. (1981), *Ethics in Nursing* (Oxford: Oxford University Press).

Bloch, M. and Parry, J. (eds), (1982) *Death and the Regeneration of Life* (Cambridge: Cambridge University Press).

Brindle, B. 1 July 1990. 'Resounding call of the whistle-blower nurse' *Guardian*.

Brindle, B. 18 August 1990. 'Managers say barred nurse lacks backing' *Guardian*.

Calabresi, G. and Bobbitt, P. (1978), *Tragic Choices* (New York: Norton).

Callanan M. and Kelley, P. (1992), *Final Gifts: Understanding and helping the dying* (London: Hodder & Stoughton).

Channon, H. (1990), 'The Team Splitter', in C. M. (ed.), *Hospice and Palliative Care: An interdisciplinary approach* (London: Edward Arnold).

Dunlop, R. J. and Hockey, J. M. (1990), *Terminal Care Support Teams: The hospital-hospice interface* (Oxford: Oxford University Press).

Gittings, C. (1984), *Death Burial and the Individual in Early Modern England* (London: Croom Helm).

Glaser, G. G. and Strauss, A. L. (1966), *Awareness of Dying* (London: Martin Robertson).

Gorer, G. (1965), *Death, Grief & Mourning* (London: Cresset Press).

Harris, M. (1990), 'Other Ethical Dilemmas', in C. M. (ed.), *Hospice and Palliative Care: An interdisciplinary approach* (London: Edward Arnold).

Hull, R., Ellis, M., Sargent V., (1989), *Teamwork in Palliative Care* (Oxford: Radcliffe Medical Press).

Illich, I. (1977), *Limits to Medicine: Medical Nemesis* (Harmondsworth, Penguin).

Jackson, L. (1990), 'Team Building', in C. M. (ed.), *Hospice and Palliative Care: An interdisciplinary approach* (London: Edward Arnold).

Kennedy, I. (1981), *The Unmasking of Medicine* (London: George Allen & Unwin).

Kellehear, A. (1984), 'Are we a "Death-Denying" Society?' *A Sociological Review Social Science & Medicine*, vol. 18, no 9, pp. 713–23.

Kubler-Ross, E. *AIDS: The Ultimate Challenge* (New York: Macmillan Publishing Company).

Lewis, J. (1986), *What Price Community Medicine?* (Brighton: Wheatsheaf.)

Lunn, L. (1993), 'Spiritual Concerns in Palliation', in Saunders, C. M. and Sykes, N. (eds) *'The Management of Terminal Malignant Disease'* (London: Edward Arnold.)

Malinowski, B., (1974), *Magic, Science & Religion* (London: Souvenir).

McKeown, T. (1979), *The Role of Medicine: Dream, mirage or nemesis?* (Oxford, Blackwell, London).

McNulty, B. J. (1978), 'Outpatient and Auxiliary Management from a Hospice' in ed Saunders, C. *The Management of Malignant Disease.* (London: Edward Arnold).

Owens, P. (1987), *Community Care and Severe Physical Disability* (London: NCVO/Bedford Square Press).

O'Brien, T. (1990), 'The Twenty-four Hours Before and After Death', in C. M. (ed.), *Hospice and Palliative Care: An interdisciplinary approach* (London: Edward Arnold).

Pritchard, E. R., Collard, J., Starr, F., Lockwood, J. A., Kutscher, A. H., and Seeland, I.B. (1979), *Home Care: Living with Dying* (New York: Columbia University Press).

Saunders, C. (1978), (ed.) *The Management of Malignant Disease* (London: Edward Arnold).

Saunders, C. M. and Sykes, N. (eds) (1993), *The Management of Terminal Malignant Disease* (London: Edward Arnold).

Saunders, C. and Baines M. (1989), *Living with Dying, the management of terminal disease* (Oxford: Oxford University Press).

Saunders, C. M. (1990), *Hospice and Palliative Care: An interdisciplinary approach* (London: Edward Arnold).

Stone, L. (1979), *Family, Sex & Marriage 1500–1800* (London: Weidenfeld & Nicolson).

The Times (1992), 'Winchester doctor to appeal before magistrates charged with attempted murder after the death of one of his patients', 8 January.

The Times (1993) 'Doctor returns to work with suspended sentence', 3 Febuary.

Turner, V. (1969), *The Ritual Process: Structure & Anti-structure* (The Times (1993) 'Docter returns to wash with suspended sentence', 3 February. Chicago: Aldine Publishing Company).

Van Gennep, A. (1965), *Rites of Passage* (London: Routledge & Kegan Paul).

West, T. (1990), 'Multidisciplinary Working', in C. M. (ed.), *Hospice and Palliative Care: An interdisciplinary approach* (London: Edward Arnold).

Wood, (1990), 'Intractable Symptoms', in C. M. (ed.), *Hospice and Palliative Care: An interdisciplinary approach* (London: Edward Arnold).

9 *Primary health care*

Margot Jefferys

Chapter summary

The author describes the development of Primary Health Care from the creation of the National Health Service until the 1980s. The division of service provision between local authorities and health services perpetuated older professional hostilities and was counter-productive to interprofessional collaboration. The changing status and power of key professional groups of doctors, nurses and social workers over time are described. Important changes and developments towards more partnership and group arrangements in general practice in the 1960s and 1970s, and NHS contractual arrangements in the 1980s and 1990s, have inevitably moved primary health care into a more teamwork-orientated approach.

Introduction

The Oxford English Dictionary tells us that the word 'team' is of Anglo-Saxon origin. An early mention of it in an English manuscript referred to oxen, yoked to carts. For many centuries apparently, it was used only to refer to animals in harness. In the eighteenth century, it was sometimes used to describe workers – or 'hands' – involved in co-ordinated tasks. By the mid-nineteenth century, with the development of organised recreational sport, the term had begun to acquire a new, more positive connotation.

By the twentieth century, as a result of the size and complexity of the typical industrial enterprise, dependent on the smooth dovetailing of the activities of individuals in many walks of life (and perhaps also of the need to emphasise common goals in war situations), individuals began to be judged on their ability to work harmoniously in teams or to lead them. Such traits began to be valued as much as those of innate intelligence or personal drive.

The advantages of teamwork, however, have been much more self-evident in task-orientated bodies which are unitary organisations.

This generally means both workplaces located in a delimited physical space – such as a factory, department store or hospital – and contractual conditions of employment which specify hierarchical lines of responsibility.

Given the location and structure of the work units which deliver the various elements of service which in the British scene we call primary health care, it is not surprising that, until comparatively recently, teams and teamwork have been more noticeable by their absence than by their presence. General practice, the bedrock of today's primary health care, is based on independent contractors, not salaried employees. Only in the last half century have they begun to work in partnerships of more than two. Only even more recently have they begun habitually to employ receptionists, secretaries and managers, let alone surgery-based nurses to assist them in their clinical work.

District or home nurses, health visitors and social workers, the other main participants in the delivery of primary health care, have always been salaried employees of bureaucratic organisations, now the local authority and the district health authority. In theory, they are members of intraprofessional teams who report to a superior officer, who in turn is responsible for their conduct to the employing authority. In practice, however, because in the main their work is domiciliary-based and case-orientated, they work alone rather than in groups and cannot easily be subjected to the scrutiny of peers, let alone superiors.

In the field of primary health care – the term defined here to mean the continuing health and social welfare care offered appropriately to needful individuals living in private households – a team must inevitably be an interprofessional one, and teamwork consist of activities carried out by more than one team member and communicated to one another. Since the different professionals are also likely to be employed by different authorities or be self-employed – as in the case of general practitioners – teamwork presents problems additional to and considerably more complex than those which confront professional workers employed by a single authority.

In this attempt to present the main features of the development of primary health care teams, I have chosen to distinguish three main, albeit overlapping, phases since the formation of the National Health Service which is my starting point. I have also tried to consider, within each phase, the particular problems facing the occupational groups which have ultimately become the principal actors in what is now commonly called the primary health care team.

The first phase runs roughly from the formation of the NHS in 1948 to the mid-1960s; the second, from then until the early 1980s; and the third, from the mid-1980s to the present time. The professional groups concerned include general practitioners and other community-based doctors; district nurses, domiciliary midwives, health visitors; and social workers of various denominations working for statutory or voluntary bodies and therapists.

The early years of the NHS

The idea of establishing a team, each member of which would have a distinctive role to play in providing a comprehensive personal health service to those living in a defined community in a particular vicinity, is not a recent one. As long ago as 1920, the Consultative Council on Medical and Allied Services, a body set up to advise the Ministry of Health, recommended, in what later became known as the Dawson Report (Dawson, 1920; Honigsbaum, 1979, pp. 64–72), that neighbourhood and preventive health services should be assembled into a single organisation – that is, that there should be a network of 'primary health centres' throughout the country. These were envisaged as incorporating general practitioners and other health and social welfare workers employed by local authorities or voluntary organisations.

The Dawson recommendations were not implemented at the time, for a variety of reasons which need not concern us here, but the idea of a primary health care centre bringing together those concerned with the health as well as the medical and nursing care of individuals living in the community was not entirely lost. It became an objective of the Socialist Medical Association which was influential, in the Second World War and immediately after it, in shaping the provisions of the National Health Service (Honigsbaum, 1979, pp. 255–66). Embodied in the 1946 Act which brought the NHS into being two years later was a clause which enabled local health authorities to set up health centres in which general practitioners could rent surgeries to conduct their medical care services, alongside the domiciliary nursing and midwifery, health visiting, school nursing and other services for which the local Health Authority itself was responsible (NHS Act, 1946: Part III, section 21).

In the event, little use was made of this statutory provision in the two decades which followed the Second World War (Webster, 1988, pp. 380–8). Local authorities had more pressing priorities, especially in the field of housing, than the construction of new buildings for public health purposes. Moreover, older general practitioners were scarcely in the mood to become local authority tenants. Many of them believed that the infant welfare and maternity services which local authorities had developed in the pre-1939 era had clandestinely treated sick mothers and children, thus depriving them of potential patients (Honigsbaum, 1979, pp. 83–5; Lindsey, 1962, pp. 20 and 366). They conveniently forgot, of course, that widespread poverty among those who attended the local authorities' clinics would have precluded many of them from paying much, if anything, for any medical treatment which they might seek.

In the new NHS, of course, mothers and children who registered with them became their patients, for which they received a per capita payment automatically whether or not they consulted; but these patients were also entitled to receive advice on infant management from health visitors who were under a statutory obligation to visit and report to the Medical Officer of Health. Health visitors, fully qualified nurses with additional training in preventive and promotive medicine, were likely to be more knowledgeable about such matters than the general practitioners who had had no such training. Hence, a potential source of conflict was perpetuated (Jefferys, 1965, pp. 312–13).

General practitioners

Unresolved, historically-based resentment of local authorities and their medical and nursing staff, however misconceived or exaggerated, was not the only reason for general practitioner unreadiness to consider close collaboration with others during the 1950s. Morale, never very high perhaps, except among a minority of prosperous, successful doctors working in more affluent areas and usually able to admit patients to and treat them in small cottage hospitals, had been severely undermined by the terms negotiated on their behalf at the formation of the NHS. On the surface, at least, the terms appeared to be very detrimental to general practitioners as compared to hospital-based specialists, including those general physicians who had acquired the coveted title of consultant and the continued right to practise privately (Lindsey, 1962, ch. VI).

General practitioners, it is true, had succeeded in retaining the status of independent contractor as against that of salaried employee, the former being essential, they claimed, to safeguard their right to clinical freedom. It was part of their claim to professional status by which they set great store, claiming superiority over those health workers, such as midwives and nurses, whose status as employees was one of subordination either to a medical officer or to an administrator. At the same time the GPs had lost the power to buy and sell practices, and the imposition of per capita payment as the main form of remuneration, fixed initially at a level which over a lifetime would reward them less well than hospital consultants, reinforced the widespread feeling among them that they had been assigned to second-class status within the new health care system (Lindsey, 1962, pp. 126–54).

Furthermore, the contracts which they felt forced to sign with the Local Executive Councils allowed little in the way of reimbursement of expenses incurred in maintaining premises or improving the quantity or quality of service which they provided. For example, those who chose to employ a practice receptionist or nurse, instead of the customary practice of using the unpaid services of a wife to act in one or both these capacities, had to do so out of their own incomes. No wonder there was little incentive for all but the most dedicated and charitable to draw other professionals closely into their work.

It was also difficult for the single-handed practitioner to realise that, with the universal provision of free access to general practice services which the NHS Act provided, the market for medical services had altered. An individual practitioner no longer had to fear that fee-paying patients would be poached from him by competitors. Nevertheless the 'cottage industry' mentality survived and served to perpetuate the isolation from and suspicion of his peers which had been a feature of the earlier history of general practice (Brotherston, 1971, pp. 85–126). This mentality was reinforced by the location from which most general practitioners worked. Considerable numbers conducted their practices from their homes. Those who did not, often used cramped, unsuitable premises such as lock-up shops in city centres.

The move to form partnerships of two or more principals – that is of co-equals – which ultimately helped to end the dysfunctional isolation, came about only gradually, leaving behind for the most part those who felt most threatened by the changes which were occurring contemporaneously in medical sciences, in technology and in societal values (Cartwright, 1967).

Medical Officers of Health

Hitherto, I have considered the factors which at the formation of the NHS prevented general practitioners from entering health centres or collaborating willingly with health professionals employed by the local authority to provide preventive, promotive and supportive community health and welfare services which would complement those provided by the general practitioners themselves. It is time now to turn to what was happening to the personnel who were beginning to provide such services and what was promoting or preventing moves on their part to become more closely involved in collaborative teamwork with other health and social welfare professionals, including general practitioners.

Local authority Medical Officers of Health, as a body, were also somewhat dismayed by the shape of the new National Health Service. Since 1929, they had been responsible for the municipal hospitals – the one-time poor law infirmaries; but in the 1946 settlement all hospitals came under the jurisdiction of new regional and local hospital boards. Their responsibilities for community-based preventive and domiciliary nursing care expanded, and most of them became Chief Medical Officers to their Local Education Authority's school health service.

Some also became Chief Welfare Officers responsible for community-based services for a range of disabled adults and children. But many of them felt they had lost status with their exclusion from hospital administration, and they suffered an additional blow when, in 1948, new legislation established local authority children's departments, which were headed by non-medically qualified officers responsible to the Home Office, not the Ministry of Health.

In these circumstances, Medical Officers of Health were also likely to be defensive and to guard jealously the authority which they felt they still retained over the multi-occupational work force under their command. The idea that the nurses, health visitors and social workers which constituted this force should work closely with general practitioners who showed little sign of valuing their activities did not immediately commend itself to most of them (Webster, 1988, p. 349).

Assistant Medical Officers – often married women employed part-time – served in the local authority infant welfare and school health clinics. They had little status within the medical profession and were sometimes regarded by general practitioners as little more than failed clinicians.

District nurses and midwives

District nurses and midwives, although employees of the Medical Officer of Health's department, for the most part took their orders directly from their nursing superior. Midwives justifiably felt themselves to be professionals in their own right and, although they were under an obligation to call in the general practitioner whose patient wished the latter to be present for a domiciliary delivery. They felt resentful of a system which rewarded the GP for attendance when it was often no more than a token appearance. District nurses took referrals from both general practitioners and hospitals; they seldom had any meaningful contact with either, although general practitioners were often fulsome in their praise of the work undertaken by district or home nurses, particularly with their elderly patients. Their records belonged to the public health department and were not integrated with the GP's own patient record.

Health visitors and social workers

Health visitors, it was widely acknowledged, had played a significant part in maintaining nutritional and hygienic standards in the interwar and war years. Yet their work in preventing what we now call child abuse came under attack in the immediate post-war years. They were deprived of legal responsibility for it in 1948 when the children's departments were established in local authorities under the auspices of the Home Office, not the Ministry of Health. There was also a challenge to the claim which had been made on their behalf that they were *par excellence* the ideal 'family visitor' able to help vulnerable families with a range of social and psychological as well as health problems. The gauntlet was thrown down by those who were pressing the need for university-trained social workers in local authority services. A working party on Health Visiting, which was set up in the 1950s and in its report endorsed the proposal, was belittled by those intent on capturing the field of family welfare for an emergent although still embryonic social work profession (Jameson, 1956).

The challenge was led by an elite group who, unlike nurses, had had a university training which emphasised psychoanalytical theory rather than pragmatic, hands-on learning. This group had begun to enter local authority employment through child guidance work in the school health service and the domiciliary mental health and welfare services as well as through the children's departments. To say that inter-occupational competition for professional territory did not create the right climate for collaboration is an understatement.

Mutual suspicion, leading to misrepresentation, denigration and hostility, characterised the divided, community-based health and social welfare services of the 1950s. Yet, at the same time, it was becoming clearer to many health and social service planners as well as to participants in all the community-based services that the tripartite structure of health services and the lack of liaison between general practitioners, hospital staff and local authority personnel was seriously reducing the quality of the services which could be delivered to patients and their families (Lindsey, 1962, p. 454).

An era of challenge – mid-1950s to mid-1980s

The impetus for far-reaching changes in the ways in which the health and welfare agencies and their personnel were to relate to one another did not come primarily from a sudden realisation of the harm which failure to co-operate did to patients or clients. The ground swell from such an impetus must not be totally discounted, but what ultimately persuaded the powers that be to facilitate change in both service structures and professional practice was their growing belief that the failure of communit-based service personnel to work together effectively was leading to an ever greater pressure for hospital admission. Hospital care was essentially expensive care, and the rapidly increasing cost – an almost uncontrollable item to be met by the tax payer. The quest for better community-based services was seen as both financially and socially desirable.

It would be a mistake to suggest that the sorry state of general practitioners, described earlier, had persisted without modification into the mid-1960s. Forward-looking GPs had already founded the College of General Practitioners in 1952 (in 1962 it acquired the prefix 'Royal'), with the specific aim of raising professional standards throughout that sector of the NHS (Fry *et al.*, 1983). The College provided a forum in which the responses which general practitioners should give to the challenges created by new disease patterns, new medical knowledge and technologies, and new social and economic circumstances affecting both them and their patients, could be debated.

Early in the 1960s, however, policy-makers began to recognise that general practice was undergoing a crisis. Few British medical graduates were choosing voluntarily to enter it, opting frequently for emigration rather than enduring the unfavourable professional conditions for practice. In so far as recruitment was maintained, it was quite often due to Asian doctors, whose primary purpose in coming to Britain was to obtain postgraduate, specialist training, filling vacant posts. After a report which set out deliberately to boost the opportunities for satisfying work in general practice (Gillie, 1963), the British Medical Association, through the General Medical Services Committee, began to negotiate with central government for better remuneration and conditions of work for the country's family doctors. By 1966, when an agreement entitled 'The Family Doctors' Charter' was reached, the Ministry of Health was well aware that an improvement in the remuneration and status of general practitioners, relative to that of hospital-based consultants, could also help to stem if not to halt the rapidly increasing relative cost of the hospital sector (BMA, 1965).

'The Family Doctors' Charter' not only helped to improve the status of general practitioners *vis-à-vis* the hospital consultant: it also included a variety of measures which had the beneficial effect of enabling the development of some degree of intraprofessional and interprofessional teamwork (Jefferys and Sachs, 1983, pp.3–5). For example, it provided allowances to general practitioners who grouped together to practise from common premises. It encouraged them to employ receptionists and practice nurses by offering reimbursement of the greater part of the salaries. It provided interest-free loans for the improvement (which often meant the enlargement) of practice premises, and more space facilitated staff meetings.

The 1960s also began to see a *rapprochement* between the two community-based sectors of the NHS. Some far-seeing Medical Officers of Health recognised that the value of the preventive, promotive and supportive services which their staffs were supposed to deliver would be greatly enhanced were those staff to work closely with their patients' general practitioners (Health Services & Public health Act, 1968, sections 10–11). They were able to persuade some of the more open-minded general practitioners in their bailiwicks to provide accommodation in their practices for the health department's health visitors, district nurses or midwives who had responsibility for the same patients. Little by little, the practice of attachment spread, so that by the mid-1970s, the majority of health visitors, for example, were 'attached' to general practice. In other words, they were responsible for individuals on a general practitioner's list and not, as before, for the residents of a district.

One other mid-1960s development also encouraged joint general practice–local authority co-operation. In 1965, official central government encouragement was given to the building of health centres by local authorities (Ministry of Health, 1965). Some younger GP principals, who had not inherited the tribal hostility to local authorities of some of their older peers, were quite willing to take up tenancies in them. In doing so, they were absolved from the necessity to make a long-term commitment to invest in the purchase of equivalently desirable premises on council estates. The advantage, besides the sharing of common premises with the local authority and possibly other GP tenants, was the availability of a range of local authority health and welfare facilities in the same building.

These changes in the structure of general practice were accompanied by a noticeable shift in the ideas about what general practice should be about among many of the most active members of the Royal College of General Practitioners. In retrospect, it is easy to recognise the great importance of the ideas supplied by Balint, a psychoanalytically orientated psychiatrist, who began to undertake group work with some practising general practitioners (Balint, 1957). He gave them a new focus for their work, and one which helped them to distinguish their role from that of hospital-based specialists in body system medicine or surgery. Moreover, the role, as he defined it, was not an inferior one. Like those of hospital specialists, it implied a unique body of knowledge; but unlike that of body system specialists it was based on a holistic view first of patients as people living in complex social relationships, and secondly of themselves as part of that social environment and hence of a relationship which, in itself, could be therapeutic or non-therapeutic.

At the time, the Balint model was fiercely contested by those GPs who considered that it jeopardised their claims to traditional clinical skills grounded in basic orthodox medical training. Rather than enhance their standing *vis-à-vis* the consultants, they feared that to accept a Balint model would be to undermine their professional status still further.

By itself, the Balint model for their future role did not offer GPs a clear, unequivocal picture of what their relationship with other community-based health and welfare professionals should be. Indeed, it suggested that GPs could and should become the competent professionals in a field which psychiatric and other trained social workers were already claiming as their own – the basis of their own unique expertise. There were grounds there for potential interprofessional conflict, particularly since the burgeoning social work profession, during the 1960s, was making a bid for increased authority in the developing personal social services of local government.

Social workers, through the Committee of Enquiry chaired by Dame Eileen Younghusband, had proposed an enlarged role for social workers in local government and set out the requisite training requirements (Younghusband, 1959). Her recommendations had been accepted at least to the extent that a Training Council was established alongside one for Health Visitors (Health Visitor & Social Work Training Act, 1962). As important was the decision by the Joseph Rowntree Memorial Fund Trust to finance a National Institute of Social Work Training in 1965 to give leadership and direction to the developing profession. In 1965, with the return of a Labour Government, a successful lobbying exercise resulted in the appointment of a Committee under the chairmanship of Frederick Seebohm (later Lord Seebohm), which was asked to prepare a plan for the development of local authority personal social services (Seebohm, 1968). It reported in 1968 and its recommendations were largely accepted and enacted in 1970, together with an Act which increased the mandate given to local government to provide a range of support services for chronically sick and disabled people.

The Seebohm programme resulted in practice in the creation of social service departments in local government into which were drawn all the non-medical personal social service workers who had hitherto been employed in the health, welfare, and education departments of the authorities. The administrative leadership of the new departments was given to directors whose appointments had to be endorsed by the Secretary of State and whose basic qualification normally was expected to be that of a university-trained social worker.

At the same time, the new departments were urged to merge their workforces into locally-based units composed of social workers with a basic two-year training, who, it was argued, would be qualified to give personal advice on all the commonly experienced social and psychological problems of disadvantaged individuals and families. The *ad hoc* specialisms which had grown up over past decades to deal with problems of special groups, such as the elderly, children, the blind, deaf and mentally disordered or retarded, were considered to have given a poor service to their clients because of the narrow focus of their training and to have encouraged either unnecessary or positively disruptive overlapping of services or unacceptable gaps.

It is easy to see in retrospect that the value of focused services as well as of having additional training for those responsible for individuals with serious psychiatric problems, was seriously underrated. So too was the scale of the demand for services which the new legislation and rising societal expectations would place upon the nascent departments. The potential too for dysfunctional disharmony between those who remained in the rump of the health departments (for example, the health visitors) and those who became part of the growing social service empires, was hardly foreseen.

Nevertheless, although the changes in the local authority structures of both the personal social services and the NHS which took place during the 1970s were disturbing to the personnel of these services and, for that reason, provided a poor basis for interprofessional trust and collaboration, the general social climate of the times was conducive to greater openness to new ideas which challenged the sacred cows that every profession had fiercely herded in defence of its own narrowly conceived professional interests.

In particular, increasing numbers of GPs demonstrated their greater self-confidence by consolidating their solo or two-person practices into groups working from greatly improved premises where the health authority's health visitors, district nurses and midwives could also find a base. In addition, more and more practitioners began to employ their own surgery nurses, who were soon able to demonstrate their capacity to undertake a range of procedures which, previously, GPs had felt obliged to perform themselves or obtain for their patients from hospitals.

This was a period too when GPs became even more adventurous. Some courted the social service departments, begging the latter to attach social workers to their practices for at least part of the working week so that they could liaise directly on tackling the infinite variety of psychological, social and economic problems displayed by their patients. Some provided accommodation and sessions for counsellors working for such voluntary organisations such as Relate, so that they could provide a better service for their patients suffering from emotional distress. Others sought regular help from physiotherapists and/or occupational therapists employed by the NHS or the local authority.

The experiences of varied forms of attachment of health and allied workers to general practices in the primary care setting were not only important in their own right. They also served indirectly to further co-operation by demonstrating to GPs that they were part of a network of services which together could help to meet their patients' needs and expectations.

The background to the contemporary scene – the 1980s

It is a trite truism to state that in human history things never stand still. The widespread desire of the professional groups involved in the developments in primary health care of the 1970s was for a period of calm consolidation: it did not materialise. The Conservative government viewed the NHS as a state monopolistic enterprise, and *ipso facto* inherently inefficient in its use of resources. Despite its popularity and the absence of pressure from inside or outside the NHS for fundamental reform, the Thatcher philosophy held that it could be vastly improved, without inviting ever more expenditure, by encouraging competition between providers at both hospital and general practice level to improve the quality of care. And so began the series of moves to impose management structures at every level of the NHS, to stimulate competition through the creation of internal markets, and to distinguish purchaser and provider roles.

Where general practice was concerned, the government hoped to achieve its policy of encouraging competition and increasing efficiency first, by affecting radical changes in the contract for GP principals (Griffiths, 1988), and secondly, by introducing a scheme whereby GP groups with more than 10,000 patients registered with them could hold their own budgets.

The new style GP contract came into force in 1990, despite considerable misgivings from the profession. Among its provisions is a requirement to provide the Family Health Services Authority, which holds their contracts, with an annual report on their activities and practice development proposals, specifying arrangements for patient access, including the hours they will be available in their surgeries. In addition, they must provide the FHSA with regular information on their preventive medicine activities (to include immunisation of children and annual, unsolicited consultations with all their registered patients aged 75 years or more). Their performance in these fields determines how much they get paid for these procedures. Those who fail to reach set targets receive minimum payments only; those who reach or surpass them are financially rewarded. The government's intention in introducing these measures is to establish the concept of performance rating in health promotion, especially for patients who fall into their priority groups.

Under the contract, the revised remuneration structure increases the per capita payments for patients and allows more to register. At the same time it reimburses a smaller proportion of the salaries of non-medical staff, such as nurses, secretaries and receptionist, employed in the practice. Previous restrictions on advertising their services to attract potential patient registrations have been largely removed. It is less complicated for patients to change their GPs if they are dissatisfied. They will no longer have to give their GP the reasons and ask for her or his permission.

The stated government objective in introducing all these measures into the new GP contract is to reintroduce an element of general practitioner competition which it considers has been missing since the NHS was founded and which, if restored, will improve the quality of primary health care services.

From 1990 also, the government's budget-holding provisions have been brought into force. GPs who wished to become budget-holders had to show that all the principals in the practice agreed. The budget is intended to cover the estimated costs of both the medicines likely to be reasonably prescribed during the year and a range of specific hospital procedures and other specialist services likely to be needed by them. These latter may be purchased from any source, either NHS or private, with whom the GP is able to negotiate a contract. In their own interests, as well as that of their patients, budget-holders are encouraged to 'shop around' to achieve the 'best buy'.

The object of these provisions was at least twofold. In the first place, it was believed that budget-holding GPs would become more aware of the cost to the NHS of their own clinical decision- making, and consequently be more circumspect in the way in which they initiated expenditure elsewhere in the system. In the second place, it was intended to provide a financial incentive to treat and/or carry out diagnostic investigations required by patients in the community rather than in the hospital. It was argued that the budget-holding scheme would, at one and the same time, be cost-effective, preferred by most patients, and professionally stimulating for the GPs who opted to hold their own budgets.

In subsequent years more GPs have become budget-holders. Those who were pioneers in this respect have for the most part been enthusiastic. Some of the more recent budget-holders have had negative reasons for joining the scheme. They believe, despite denials from managers of Trust or non-Trust hospitals, that patients registered with budget-holders have been given greater priority for admission from hospital waiting lists than those of non-budgetholders.

It is not possible at the time of writing to gauge the effect, if any, of the 1990 GP contract or of budget-holding, on teams or teamwork in primary health care. The emphasis on intraprofessional competition for patient numbers and allegiance is interpreted by some as a regressive return to the pre-Second World War era when mutual suspicion among GP was rife and accusations of patient-pinching frequent. On the other hand, even some of those who are dismayed by the new ideological ambience affecting health service delivery grudgingly admit that some of the new measures have the potential for improving the quality of the services provided by and in general practice. The new contract, in particular, shifts the balance of general practice work, if only marginally, towards disease and disability prevention and positive health promotion. In so doing, it is likely to persuade many GPs that these tasks can be most easily carried out in conjunction with other health professionals for whom such tasks are central.

Parallel developments in community social welfare provision

The NHS is not the only major public sector enterprise to be put through a process of re-evaluation in the 1980s. Successive Thatcher governments were particularly critical of local government bodies, especially if they were dominated by their political opponents. The government's policy was to restrict their powers and to impose national norms for the services for which local government was responsible.

Here it faced, however, a dilemma. The number and proportion of very old individuals in the population was increasing and with it the pressure on health and social support services of all kinds. At the same time, the expectations of individuals for better health and higher standards of social welfare were rising as a result of innovations in medical technology, taking place mainly in the expensive hospital sector. They were not only demonstrably saving life but helping to improve its quality. Hip replacements and pacemakers are classic examples of the latter. All these factors placed pressures on governments to increase expenditure on health and welfare services.

For ideological reasons the government was not anxious to assign the task of providing a better range of community social welfare services for elderly frail and/or disabled individuals to local authorities. It had hoped that Griffiths, a successful business executive who had earlier proposed a new management structure for the NHS, would be able to suggest a new agency outside local government to take charge of the administration of arrangements to meet the needs in the community of the growing numbers of elderly people as well as of physically disabled and mentally disordered individuals and those with learning difficulties.

In the event, after exploring many options, Griffiths considered that social services departments were the appropriate agencies and recommended as much to the government. After a considerable delay, occasioned, it has been alleged, by the reluctance of the Conservative government to entrust local government with the mammoth task, the major Griffith recommendations were embedded in the NHS and Community Care Act of 1990. The provisions for community care came into operation in April 1993. Local authorities receive resources which, up to that date, had been dispensed by central government through the Department of Social Security.

'Care managers' appointed by the social service departments are authorised to work out individualised packages of care after discussion with the clients themselves, their caring relatives and the responsible health and social service personnel – which may include district nurses, social workers and others as well as the GP.

It is too early at the time of writing to assess the effects of the implementation of this new legislation on teamwork in primary care settings. There are grounds for disquiet, if not for grim foreboding, at a time when the favoured managerial ethos for the NHS as well as for local government social services appears to concentrate on competition, efficiency and rationing rather than on collaboration. However, if the objectives of the community care provisions of the Act do not remain empty rhetoric, there should be much greater emphasis than there was in the past on drawing the intended recipients of services and their significant carers into the primary health care team and the decision-making and monitoring process. Such involvement, if it occurs on a general scale, cannot but mark an important advance in the practice as well as the theory of teamwork in primary health care.

References

Balint, M. (1957), *The Doctor, His Patient and the Illness* (London: Pitman, second edn).

British Medical Association (1965), *A Charter for the Family Doctor Service* (London: BMA).

Brotherston, J. H. F. (1971), 'The Evolution of Medical Practice', in G. McLachlan and T. McKeown (eds), *Medical History and Medical Care* (London: Oxford University Press).

Cartwright, A. (1967), *Patients and their Doctors* (London: Routledge & Kegan Paul).

Dawson Report (1920), *Interim Report of the Consultative Council on Medical and Allied Services* (London: HMSO).

Fry, J., Hunt, Lord and Pinsent, R. J. F. H. (1983), *A History of the Royal College of General Practitioners* (Lancaster: M. T. P. Press).

Gillie, A. (Chairman) (1963), *The Field of Work of the Family Doctor*, Report from the Standing Medical Advisory Committee of the Central Health Services Council (London: HMSO).

Griffiths, R. (1988), *Community Care. An Agenda for Action* (London: HMSO).

Health Services & Public Health Act, 1968 (London: HMSO).

Health Visitor and Social Working Training Act, 1962 (London: HMSO).

Honigsbaum, F. (1979), *The Division in British Medicine* (London: Kegan Paul).

Jameson, W. (Chairman) (1956), *An Enquiry into Health Visiting,* Report of a Ministry of Health Working Party (London: HMSO).

Jefferys, M. (1965), *An Anatomy of Social Services* (London: Michael Joseph).

Jefferys, M. and Sachs, H. (1983), *Rethinking General Practice* (London: Tavistock Press).

Lindsey, A. (1962), *Socialized Medicine in England & Wales* (Chapel Hill. NC: University of N. Carolina Press).

Ministry of Health (1959), Circular HM(65) no. 25 (London: HMSO).

National Health Service Act, 1946 (London: HMSO).

Seebohm, F. (Chairman) (1968), *Local Authority and Allied Personal Social Services* Report of Ministry of Health's Committee, Cmnd 3703 (London: HMSO).

Webster, C. (1988), *Health Services since the War* (London: HMSO).

Younghusband, E. (Chairman) (1959), *Social Workers in Local Authority Health & Welfare Services.* Report of Ministry of Health Working Party (London: HMSO).

SECTION THREE
Inside teamwork

10 *Learning to work effectively in teams*

Peter Pritchard

Chapter summary

This chapter provides a framework for action. The author sets out the theoretical background to teamwork, and strategies for developing successful interprofessional work. It readdressess many of the questions that have been raised in earlier chapters about professional roles, status and hierarchy, and the development of common organisational objectives. The characteristics of successful teams are discussed and analysed with reference to particular initiatives and a variety of educational techniques, including the role of facilitators in bringing about organisational change.

Introduction

Can we learn to work effectively in teams?

To put a group of doctors and nurses together in an operating theatre and expect them to undertake brain surgery, without joint training, would be unrealistic. Yet that has been the traditional approach to primary health care (PHC) teams. The team members may be very skilled at their own jobs, but few have received any education or training in how to work together as an effective team.

Teamwork is not a mysterious black art for which training is long and difficult. The basic requirements for effective teamwork were studied at the Massachusetts Institute of Technology in the early 1970s (Beckhard, 1972; Rubin and Beckhard, 1972), using action-research techniques based on organisational psychology. Their methods have been tried and evaluated in a number of settings in many countries. Until lately, however, there has been reluctance in the UK to invest in team development.

The need for effective team working is widely accepted, particularly as general practice tries to develop more preventive and health promotive strategies. The implementation of the Community Care Act in April 1993 (Secretary of State for Health, 1990), has reinforced the need for teamwork (see Jefferys, ch. 9). Fortunately, major team development initiatives are now under way, and research into the effectiveness of teamwork is being undertaken in several centres.

This chapter aims to look first at teamwork in primary health care – what it is and what it does – and then to consider ways of helping teams to operate effectively for the benefit of the public, as well as the professional and lay people involved.

What is a team?

Definition and essential characteristics

A definition of a team (Rubin and Beckhard, 1972; Gilmore *et al.*, 1974, pp. 5–6) which has stood the test of time is:

> A team is a group of people who make different contributions towards the achievement of a common goal

These authors go on to describe the essential characteristics of teamwork, based on seven literature sources between 1956 and 1968, as follows (slightly paraphrased):

- The members of a team share a common purpose which binds them together and guides their actions.
- Each member of the team has a clear understanding of his or her own functions, appreciates and understands the contribution of the other professions in the team and recognises common interests and skills.
- The team works by pooling knowledge, skills and resources and all members share responsibility for the outcome of their decisions.
- The effectiveness of a team is related to its capability to carry out its work and to manage itself as an interdependent group of people.

These four statements are fundamental to effective team operation, and will be addressed in later sections. Bruce (1980) commented further: 'An essential ingredient in the effectiveness of teamwork is the extent to which team members are willing to subordinate their own interests to the shared interest of the team.' Although this subordination of personal interests involves discipline and some loss of individual freedom, there are substantial rewards for working in an effective team, both in the potential for personal fulfilment and development, and in benefit for the patient or client.

Co-operation within the team

Bruce (1980) concluded, from research studies of teamwork, that co-operation between professionals does not necessarily follow from proximity of working or from being involved with the same client:

> It appeared to develop step by step as the frequency of contacts increased, as the relevance of such contacts increased, as a better understanding of roles emerged, accompanied by a disappearance of stereotypes, as social proximity increased, as mutual trust began to grow and problems o confidentiality to decrease.

Bruce described three modes of co-operation, 'nominal', 'convenient' and 'committed', as 'syndromes' with symptoms and signs, along the continuum from zero to total co-operation. A summary of these syndromes appears in Table 10.1 below. The author has found this table useful as a diagnostic tool in team development. However, this progression towards committed teamwork described by Bruce depends on a learning process that may need help. Otherwise many teams will remain fixed in 'nominal' or 'convenient' mode, as is sadly the picture from many studies (Hockey and Buttimore, 1970; Gregson *et al.*, 1991).

'Nominal' teamwork

This is not really team working at all. That so many of the elements of nominal co-operation exist in practice is a reflection of earlier thinking that attaching nurses to general practice would automatically result in teamwork. Attachment may be a precondition (Gregson *et al.*, 1991), but active team building is still needed.

'Convenient' teamwork

This is an extension of the handmaiden role of nurses and other (usually female) staff in PHC. The general practitioner delegates work to other staff who receive less pay. Marsh (1991) justified this on economic grounds as saving the doctor's time. That does not fit the definition of a team sharing tasks by agreement between autonomous professionals. Rather it represents the old-fashioned hierarchical business model, in which employees of lower status do as they are told.

Table 10.1   *Team co-operation*

Co-operation in:	'Nominal'	'Convenient'	'Committed'
Team goal-setting	no explicit goals	follow doctors' goals	shared explicit goals
Role percep-tions	stereotypes common	some understanding	roles clearly understood
Professional status	wide differences	differences inhibit co-operation	differences ignored
Referral of patients	to agency not to individual professional	referral by delegation	easy two-way referral, and open access
Interaction within team	very little and irregular	some inter-action	close regular interaction, formal and informal
Mutual trust	lacking	guarded	strong and developing
Communication failure	often	sometimes	exceptional
Confidentiality	a problem	problems partly solved	not a problem
Advice to patients	inconsistent	poor co-ordination	consistent
Preventive care	not possible	possible	optimum conditions

Source: modified from Bruce, N. (1980) Teamwork for Prevention (*Chichester:* John Wiley).

'Committed' teamwork

This appears as the ideal, but we must first ensure that PHC staff are prepared to accept the level of commitment that this implies. If teamwork does not enrich their work and encourage their personal development, why should they commit themselves? General practitioners can only expect other team members to show commitment to the PHC team if they do so themselves, by investing their time and energy in team co-operation and development. Where this commitment is not present, an initial educational process will be needed to change attitudes and to convince doctors and other key staff that co-operation is beneficial. Ensuring that teamwork is both effective and committed will enhance morale and motivation, and so get the flywheel turning.

Team diagnosis

Deciding where a team lies on the scale described in Table 10.1 is complex, as so many factors may be operating. Does an effective team require perfection in every category, or is it enough to have a 'critical mass' of positive factors, enough to motivate the team towards full effectiveness? As well as the point on the scale, we must consider the direction and rate of movement. For example, a team may have nearly all the criteria for effectiveness, but morale and motivation may be falling. This fall-off may take some time to manifest itself in patient outcomes, but if it is spotted early, remedial action can be sought.

Team diagnosis is an important starting point for team development. Table 10.1 may be used as a diagnostic tool by asking all team members to mark one column for each category (in confidence), then collect and tot up the totals in each column. Categories that score high or low can give an indication of the strengths and weaknesses of the team. An alternative diagnostic instrument is described by Pritchard and Pritchard (1992), based on those of Rubin *et al.* (1975). The categories are listed below:

- **Team goals** – why are we here as a team?
- **My job** (role) – who does what?
- **Procedures** – participation
  – decision-making
  – managing conflict
- **What it feels like to work here**
  – availability
  – mutual support
  – feeling of value

The first diagnostic question about goals appears as an example in Figure 10.1.

Figure 10.1   CONFIDENTIAL QUESTIONNAIRE ON TEAM WORKING-PART 1

1. Team goals

Please read both statements, and ring one letter which seems closest to the way your team functions:

Statement I 'I often wonder why we work as a team. We seem to spend a lot of time and energy doing things which I do not think important, rather than concentrating on things which help us to achieve our main goals.'

- a. Just like statement I
- b. More like I than II
- c. In between I and II
- d. More like II than I
- e. Just like statement II

Statement II 'I am very clear about what our team is trying to achieve, and we all put our efforts into it. Whenever a question arises about what needs doing we are able to get our priorities right by referring back to our main goals.'

Describe below any examples of situations in your team which illustrate your response to this question:

. . . .
. . . .
. . . .

(Source: Pritchard, P. and Pritchard, J. (1992), *Developing teamwork in primary health care: a practical workbook*, Oxford University Press [reproduced by permission]).

Why work in teams? Who benefits?

Increasing diversity of roles and tasks

Much of a doctor's or nurse's time in PHC is spent alone with the patient, and this is a feature that patients value highly. However, many of the important activities within PHC such as maternity care, the care of patients with diabetes or needing home nursing, are obvious candidates for teamwork. In addition, the focus of general practice is changing from disease-orientation to a wider appreciation of those determinants of ill health that stem from the individual's lifestyle, and the complex physical and psychosocial environment of today. This should bring GPs closer to health visitors and social workers who already have this orientation. Trends towards more care outside hospital, and increasing numbers of elderly people reinforce the need for effective and wider teamwork.

Need for objective evaluation

Effectiveness is an essential criterion, and though we can describe factors that help or hinder effectiveness, its actual measurement is elusive. Accurate data are lacking about outcomes for patients, carers (and for staff), resources used, and the achievement of goals. Few objective evaluations have been undertaken of the benefits of teamwork over individual care, nor are the boundaries of teamwork clear. Intuitively, people working in teams justify teamwork with reasons such as those listed below (from various sources):

- Care given by a group is greater than the sum of individual care.
- Rare skills are used more appropriately.
- Team working encourages continuity of care.
- The patient gets more efficient and understanding treatment when ill.
- Peer influence and informal learning within the group raise the standards of care in the community.
- Team members have greater job satisfaction and are better able to cope with failure.
- Team working co-ordinates preventive with curative work.
- Team working enhances preventive and promotive work in PHC.

These statements are difficult to confirm unless we have measurable criteria, and find out to what extent we achieve our goals.

Possible measures of effectiveness

Much thought has been given to the question of how best to evaluate the effectiveness of teamwork, but research has been scanty. Until we have valid measures of the outcome and effectiveness of teamwork, research into the structural and process factors that might contribute to it have less value. The early work on team development has been evaluated in the field (for example, Tichy, 1977). Outcome studies of teamwork are now being undertaken in several centres, so that valid measures of the quality of teamwork should soon be available (see 'issues for research and development of teamwork', p.228 below).

Different kinds of team

Three levels of teamwork

When people talk or write about PHC teamwork in UK, they mostly describe regular meetings of the whole team, though casual contacts are also favoured. The structure of teamwork described below arose from a team development exercise involving eight 'organisation development' consultants, each attached to a practice team over a period of six months, with the aim of improving teamwork in the Oxford Region. Traditional models of task-orientated teamwork did not seem to reflect reality, and the following classification was developed (Pritchard, 1981; Pritchard *et al.*, 1984).

The patient-centred, 'intrinsic' or essential team

When, for example, an elderly lady living at home with her daughter, develops a stroke, the daughter telephones the health centre or surgery, and speaks to the receptionist, who promises to tell the doctor who will visit after morning surgery. They are a team with a shared goal and task, consisting of the patient, the carer and the receptionist (and by inference, the GP who sanctions the receptionist to control his or her time). The GP then visits the home, makes a medical diagnosis and all agree that the patient should stay at home. The district nurse is asked to visit and make an assessment. They meet to agree a care plan. By now the team consists of the patient, the carer, the district nurse and the GP. As time passes, the composition of the intrinsic team may change. Information could be exchanged at the daily 'coffee-time' meeting, or when the opportunity arises.

The task-orientated, 'functional' team

At any moment, a GP and a district nurse may share ten to twenty patients being nursed at home. From time to time this mutual caseload could be reviewed, information shared, and care plans changed as needed. This is an essential part of the audit process. In the author's experience, a meeting to review the home nursing function (cases, policies and procedures) needed to take place every six weeks, and lasted half to one hour. Both parties agreed they were well worthwhile. Other team meetings were needed to review functions such as, practice nursing, health promotion and preventive medicine, social work, practice management/finance, and patient services. In a small practice, a weekly team meeting, a monthly meeting of partners and manager, and a meeting with patients about three times a year might suffice. In larger practices, one partner might co-ordinate each of the functions listed.

The organisation-orientated 'full' team

Nearly all team tasks and communication could be covered by the intrinsic and functional teams and casual meetings, backed up by a reliable message system. However, there would be some matters that affect all team members, such as projects involving major change, holiday rotas, educational activities and parties. A meeting of the full team would be needed, but these could be infrequent and brisk, because team time is costly. Frustration with irrelevant agenda items gives large team meetings a bad name. A three-level system of organising teamwork, as described here, has the potential to involve patients, both at the level of the individual sick person and at the level of the whole organisation. As in almost every other aspect of PHC teamwork, objective evaluation is missing.

Organisational issues

The PHC team and community networks

Primary health care and social work teams are only two of many caring agencies in the community. Self-care by individuals, self-help groups, voluntary agencies and approved alternative therapists, all make essential contributions to health and well-being in the community. The PHC team is in a good position to inform patients about what services are available, and to co-ordinate these activities for a patient. To achieve this needs a knowledge of the networks and agencies operating in the community. It is beyond the wit of anyone to know about them all, as there are around 800 self-help groups related to health in any one district (Knight and Gann, 1988). One function of teamwork is to pool this knowledge of helping agencies. A patient participation group can also provide much information. Some practices have employed a voluntary services organiser. The need to make full use of community networks will be heightened by the move towards more care in the community and increasing numbers of dependant elderly people.

Task or process orientated teamwork – or both?

The research workers at the Massachusetts Institute of Technology developed and tested a schema for team development. They first considered goals and tasks, then the roles of team members, then procedures for team co-operation and communication, and finally, interpersonal relationships.

An alternative approach has been to look first at team processes, such as co-operation/conflict and interpersonal relationships – more in the style of a therapeutic or 'Balint' group. Such team development may be therapeutic to group members and this is necessary when conflict is severe or the team has suffered trauma. However, without the orientation towards tasks and goas, this method may not be so efective in dealing with patients' problems. These two approaches represent a major cultural divide between the more pragmatic and goal-seeking approach of many GPs and nurses, and a more psychodynamic orientation that appeals to some GPs and social workers. Each approach has its place in teamwork. Goals are not achieved by faulty processes, so both are needed. Team diagnosis will help members to decide when to apply which method.

Teams outside primary health care

General practitioners and others working full-time from the same premises will naturally view their own team as the central one. Professionals, such as social workers, whose main place of work is outside the PHC building, may be less committed to the PHC team. They have their own teams to which their primary loyalty is directed. Co-operation between disparate teams is possible though difficult. Part-time attachment of a social worker to the PHC team, and occasional attendance by PHC team members at case conferences are not a substitute for teamwork. Much will depend upon the extent to which both groups see co-operation as important and worth the time and effort that it takes.

The Seebohm Report (1968) envisaged much closer co-operation, but the later Barclay report (1982) scarcely mentioned it at all. The situation is now changing radically as a result of the Community Care Act (Secretary of State for Health, 1990), increasing numbers of elderly and mentally ill people receiving care outside hospital. Closer co-operation will be essential, but how can mutual trust and esteem be built up as a basis for teamwork?

Shared care with hospitals

Many patients require shared care by the PHC team and a hospital team. This is particularly evident in mental health, maternity care, surgery, cancer and diabetes. Some hospital departments, frustrated by the difficulty of co-operating with GPs, employ their own liaison nurses to work in the community, but separate from the PHC team. If their role is teaching and liaison, then the technical standards of the PHC can be raised and communication enhanced. If, however, they work in isolation, there is a danger of transfer of PHC functions to hospitals, with severe problems of communication and personal responsibility. The aim of shared care is important, and attention needs to be given to this complex variety of teamwork.

Size of teams

There is a limit to the number of people who can communicate closely enough to co-ordinate their work effectively. Organisations that are too large, either become ineffective or have to spend an inordinate amount of time communicating. Belbin (1981) regards a team of ten as too large for effective decision-making, and suggests six as an ideal size. A primary health care team could only achieve this in a partnership of two or three doctors. Teams of twenty or more run into serious problems. A partnership of five doctors could have ten employed staff, and almost as many attached staff. During a one-hour meeting, each could only expect to speak for 2.4 minutes. In the event, some team members would speak for longer, so several would not be heard.

One way round the size problem is to do most of the team communication one-to-one, or in the intrinsic or functional teams, which need not exceed ten. Only the full team meeting would be oversize, and that could be carefully structured and led.

Another option is for the practice to split into 'firms', each with its own separate staff, sharing only the practice manager. This has been taken to its logical conclusion in some health centres in Iceland and

Sweden, where one GP and one nurse work as a separate unit in a suite of rooms with their (computer- held) personal list of patients. In Iceland, the nurse combines the functions of practice nurse, home nurse and public health nurse (health visitor), so continuity of care is maximised. This 'cell' system, in the author's view, works extremely well. It is compatible with team working with the rarer team members, such as the midwife, social worker, physiotherapist or diabetic care nurse. This represents a good example of the 'small is beautiful' approach, with small teams working in a larger centre.

Though small team size is imperative, larger groupings have certain advantages. For example, in a larger centre, specialised staff such as a psychologist and physiotherapist can be employed. Sessions by visiting hospital specialists can be cost-effective, and expensive technology such as laboratory and X-ray facilities can be better justified. Working under one roof, staff members themselves may feel less isolated, giving each other professional support. Above a critical size, patients/clients are more likely to find the service they need on a 'one door' basis.

Turbulent change in the environment

Health and social services are subject to internal upheavals as never before, yet have to respond to an increasingly turbulent and changing medical and social environment. New diseases, new technology, new social trends, and demographic changes all combine to make planning and evaluation of services much more difficult. Providers of health care need to be on their toes, to respond rapidly to this turbulence, likened by management writers to canoeing through 'white water' rapids.

There must be an ultimate goal, but many of the determinants of success are not under the control of the team or its members. Advantage must be taken of favourable currents, and contrary forces avoided where possible. This more opportunistic approach does not make teamwork any easier, but it certainly increases the need for effective teamwork, and the building of trust between team members, who may have to take short cuts in their normal procedures of consultation and consensus.

The time dimension

Shortage of resources and increased and unpredictable demand all impose constraints on the time available both to do one's professional work and to maintain relationships and teamwork. Shortage of time, like shortage of money, is often quoted as an excuse for inaction, whereas they could be a spur to manage time (and money) more effectively and economically. How much time do we waste? How much is effort duplicated? Do we order our priorities strictly, with regard to the urgency of action and the importance of the activity? Can we assess our personal 'time-effectiveness'?

Different professional workers have different perceptions of time and of urgency, and this can be a source of conflict in teams. General practitioners suffer from 'fractured time' (Huntington, 1981a) which gives them a sense that everything is urgent. It is a signpost to the burnout syndrome (Cooper and Hingley, 1988). This exaggerated sense of urgency may not be shared by other professionals who are not so subject to interruption, or who manage their time better.

The length of time that different professionals stay in post is relevant to teamwork. General practitioners stay for most of their career in one location. Community nurses may also stay for many years. Though difficult to quantify, there is a strong impression that social workers move on to other posts much more rapidly. The time spent in an area enhances the depth of knowledge of local people and networks, and the more transient team members may suffer a loss of confidence and commitment. The importance of this 'knowledge of familiarity' has been stressed by Göranzon and colleagues (1993).

Team members have to take time away from their main activity in order to communicate and ensure that the team works well. 'Team time' can be used more effectively if team size is small, if procedures are brisk and efficient, and meetings kept to a minimum. Unpunctuality and faulty leadership have no place in teamwork.

Some team development initiatives

Teamwork for prevention and health promotion

The need for teamwork has, in the past, been emphasised in various Government policy documents (DHSS, 1981) and in publications by the Royal College of General Practitioners (Jones, 1986). The 1990 general practitioner contract (Department of Health, 1989) laid a duty upon GPs to undertake prevention, and there has been considerable activity in this field. These new activities have placed a burden on team members, particularly practice nurses. Resulting health gain by patients has been hard to assess in the short term, though some process measures have shown an improvement, for example the uptake of cervical screening and immunisation.

The Health Education Authority (HEA) initiative

The HEA accepted the need for team development and its evaluation. Its Primary Health Care unit undertook an extensive programme of workshops. An evaluation exercise (Spratley, 1989) studied eighteen workshops held up to the end of September 1989, involving 521 PHC professionals and 122 PHC teams. Outcomes were very positive, for example:

- The workshops gave PHC teams the opportunity to reflect on their current activities, and develop plans and strategies for health promotion.
- The workshops enhanced communication, teamwork and practice organisation.
- Participants developed an increased awareness of the potential for multidisciplinary approaches to their work.
- All participating teams had developed plans for prevention and health promotion.
- Participants appreciated the emphasis placed on the value and expertise of each member of the team.
- Plans demonstrated an awareness of the need to evaluate their activities in the short, medium and longer term.
- Participants developed opportunities to involve the public in prevention and promotion, and to encourage feedback from them.
- Collaboration with other community agencies had improved.
- Workshops had clarified the kind of support that PHC teams would need for development of their plans.

A second report (Spratley, 1990) evaluated the work of nine Local Organising Teams (LOTs) up to the end of October 1990. She found that LOTs had developed an effective mechanism for disseminating the HEA workshop strategy from national to local level by devolving the initiative to local networks. Collaboration between agencies concerned with teamwork, such as Regional, District, and Family Health Service Authorities, had been considerably enhanced. Some joint planning had been undertaken. LOTs had been successful in running and evaluating workshops for primary health care teams at local level.

These workshops have helped PHC teams to enhance team working and communication, and develop plans and strategies for prevention and health promotion. The measures were mainly subjective, but there is little doubt that the HEA has made a striking contribution to the development of PHC teamwork. Evaluation over time will show whether outcomes have been positive, and health gain has ensued.

More recent figures from 1988 up to the end of 1992 (Bellew, B. personal communication), have recorded 28 LOT (planning) workshops, involving 104 teams, with 682 participants. Between 1987 and the end of 1992 there have been 219 PHC team workshops, involving 1092 teams and 5853 participants (see Table 10.3). The response to the workshops was very positive, and the initiative is spreading through local groups and networks. For many teams this has provided an awareness of the potential for teamwork, which they then followed up by a variety of methods, considered later. General practitioners have shown considerable commitment to attending these workshops, and are represented in all the LOT groups. Numbers attending PHC team workshops from the various professional groups are shown in Table 10.2.

Table 10.2   *Occupation of participants in HEA PHCT workshops*

General Practitioner	1244
Practice nurse	1035
Health visitor	847
Receptionist	769
Practice manager	713
District nurse	654
Midwife	113
Secretary	88
Community psychiatric nurse	51
Social worker	44
Others	295
Total	5853

Source: HEA PHC Unit, Oxford.

Having attended a workshop, the next stage for members of a PHC team is to set up health promotion and preventive activities in line with national guidelines, for example in the 'Health of the Nation' report (Secretary of State for Health, 1992). This is now happening, and facilitators have played an important part, many of them jointly funded in association with LOT initiatives. Many teams have arranged 'away days' for their own staff, both employed and attached, and have started to develop 'in house' learning and action. This takes time, and is not easy to evaluate. Patience, and confidence in the HEA and LOT approach, are needed until objective measures of improved team performance and health gain appear.

Evaluation of the effectiveness of teamwork is being undertaken at the MRC/ESRC Social and Applied Psychology Unit in Sheffield (Poulton and West, 1993). These workers are measuring the *viability* of the teams in terms of sustaining good enough relationships to keep working together, and *team performance* (achievement of desired outcomes) pre-workshop and post-workshop. The effectiveness of the team will be measured through self-assessment, patient satisfaction and meeting targets for health promotion set by Family Health Service Authorities (FHSAs).

West (1990) has stressed the importance of innovativeness in team effectivenes. He suggested four team factors that were centrally important:

- Team members have a shared vision and objectives
- 'Participative safety', including valuing each other's contribution and sharing information
- Commitment to excellence, with emphasis on individual and team accountability
- Innovation is strongly supported, with emphasis on new ideas and ways of working, and professional development.

This approach ties in well with Argyris and Schön's (1978) concept of 'the learning organisation' considered later, and with the principles of good practice management.

A team manifesto

The DHSS (1986) Community Nursing Review (Cumberlege Report) recommended that teams should have a written agreement about shared objectives and an understanding of mutual roles. The idea has been taken a step further in a 'primary health care team manifesto' (Adelaide Medical Centre, 1991). This document had three aims, agreed by the team: 'to provide an exemplary primary health care service; to work together as a team; and to educate ourselves, our patients, our colleagues, trainees and students from any discipline'.

These broad aims were amplified in a series of forty-three objectives, grouped under ten headings – acute care, prescribing, women's health, health promotion/preventive care, chronic care, terminal care, patient relations, teamwork, teaching and finally, audit and information systems. This agreement took two years of hard work to formalise, and can be seen as a major achievement for the team, from which many benefits can start to flow in the longer term. A strategic plan for the team, and an upgraded management structure were two examples.

A manifesto such as this could be a starting point for teams who have the will to improve. They could then decide upon their own aims and objectives. A feature of the manifesto was that the team saw itself as a learning organisation (Argyris, 1993). Patients did not seem to have any direct involvement in the exercise, and there was no mention of a team-building programme. The team's ready acceptance of cross-disciplinary student attachments might need negotiating with patients, as discussed later. These comments are not intended as criticism of this remarkable initiative.

Management issues

Can practices manage to change?

General practices are like independent businesses and not subject to hierarchical managerial control. However, the newly constituted FHSAs have far greater powers to influence general practice, and many have taken the initiative, with the help of medical and other advisers, and Medical Audit Advisory Groups (MAAGs). Many practices where teamwork is underdeveloped have major difficulties in management of the practice as a whole. Goals are not set, planning is rudimentary and crisis management is the order of the day. These practices are not capable of changing in the direction that they or the FHSA would like to go. To develop teamwork in isolation from other aspects of management is unlikely to succeed. In this situation, a broadly-based 'helping hand' approach is more acceptable than applying pressure or even offering financial incentives.

The impact of facilitators

Many FHSA general managers have accepted that health promotion needs effective team development if they are to manage change. Some FHSAs have appointed facilitators, with a wide range of tasks.

Allsop (1990) reviewed the work of facilitators as agents of change. They had many functions, depending upon their skills, context and remit. She concluded that they represented an effective and economical option for achieving change in primary health care.

There is now a National Facilitator Development Project and an Association of Practice Facilitators with over 250 members. A questionnaire study of 229 facilitators in 1992 (Bostock, 1992) produced 137 replies (60 per cent). The aims were to assess facilitators' views of their present and future role and to analyse the support and training that they needed. A summary of key points is listed below:

- Health promotion, training and team-building were major activities.
- On average, they were involved in twelve work topic areas and their roles and responsibilities were expanding.
- They were mostly 'self-starters' and self-monitors, with some managerial support.
- Less than half felt themselves to be well supported: one-third poorly supported.
- Need for further training was expressed, particularly in managing change; team-building; computer literacy; and skills in facilitation, training, group work, communication and assertiveness.
- The need for recognition of their role by accreditation was seen by two-thirds of respondents, as was the lack of a career structure.

Facilitators, many of them nurses, have a difficult role as catalysts of change. They have a demanding and unpredictable role, requiring specific training and experience. They have little or no power to ensure that GPs will listen to them, and they need to convince members of the PHC team that they are there to help, not to control or criticise.

From policies to action

The route from central policies to action in the field that leads to health gain, is a long and tortuous one, with many alternative pathways and dead ends. So far, there has been emphasis on the HEA initiative, which, in the author's view, has been outstandingly successful to date. Though the focus has been on a 'vertical' programme for developing teamwork in one area such as health promotion, the effect has been to strengthen the team in a 'horizontal' manner, so that it can be competent in many areas such as management, clinical audit, continuing clinical education and the application of information technology. The experience from the World Health Organization would favour the development of multi-purpose teams.

Learning issues

Options and levels for learning to work as a team

Learning to work as a team has many facets, ranging from understanding other professionals' values and roles, to communicating on the job. Some methods of education for teamwork are described below, starting with basic and postbasic training. At higher educational levels, goals may be remote, but mutual understanding and communication could be fostered. At the workplace, the problems can become acute and personal. Educational methods, appropriate to the setting, will be needed. This is congruent with current thinking about context-based learning (Holm and Coles, 1993).

Basic and postbasic interdisciplinary training

The notion that medical students, nurses, social workers and other health professionals should share a core curriculum of relevant topics is appealing. At postbasic level, there are many opportunities for students to become familiar with other disciplines, with visiting lecturers, joint topic-based seminars, and visits or placements in the field. Student placements in field settings are the norm in postbasic training, and the placement sites have to be approved. The CAIPE (1988) National Survey identified 695 examples of interprofessional education in the UK involving 466 agencies. Nearly all were at postbasic level, and involved district nurses and/or health visitors. Social workers were involved in half the activities, and general practitioners in one-third. The multidisciplinary element figured prominently in the educational objectives of about one-half of the initiatives.

In the case of vocational training for general practice, teaching practices have to be assessed by strict criteria before approval is given. The quality of teamwork would normally be included (RCGP, 1985). Application of these criteria has been very successful in raising standards of practice, and might do the same for teamwork. However, there is little knowledge of what these criteria are, nor whether interdisciplinary learning is effectively achieved or just exists in name.

In the PHC team setting, the GP trainee normally spends time with the district nurse, the health visitor, the practice nurse, and the practice manager. Sometimes, the social worker will accept a GP trainee during casework and for case conferences, but this is not always free of problems, not least the attitudes of the patients or clients. When the topic was discussed at length in a patient participation group (Pritchard, 1993), a clear message was received that students were acceptable when sitting in with their own discipline (for example, the GP student with the GP, and the health visitor student with the health visitor), but they firmly resisted the idea of a nurse or social work student sitting in with the doctor during a consultation. These negative attitudes could be changed in time, but do professionals have a mandate to override what their patients or clients regard as acceptable practice? The one-to-one consultation is highly valued by the public, and a sensitive approach is needed to reconcile the needs of teaching with public concerns. These constraints need not apply in team meetings where students could learn about the practicalities and dynamics of teamwork. Students would benefit even more from becoming involved in team development exercises, where these exist. The eventual aim might be that only settings which are actively involved in team development would be acceptable for student placement.

Residential workshops for members of several teams

The HEA team workshops (described earlier) are a good example. The LOT workshops represent an essential intermediate stage to get things started and provide support. They give teams the stimulus to work together on a specific task, and then follow this through when they get back to their practice. There are difficulties. First, it is impossible to get the whole team to a mid-week residential workshop, so the returning enthusiasts may provoke opposition, until all have attended. Secondly, it is difficult to sustain work on goals and tasks, and workshops may concentrate instead on improving processes such as communication. This may be an essential bridge-building exercise for some teams, before they can get down to tasks. Thirdly, the different teams attending a joint workshop may be operating at very different levels of competence, and so may have very different learning needs and rates.

The HEA workshops have been very successful in engaging the interest of many professions and agencies in the need for improved teamwork, and pointing the way forward. The enthusiasm and energy shown by LOT groups and the team workshops must be a favourable sign for the future.

'Away days' for single teams

Teams that are functioning reasonably well and are motivated to improve their performance may gain great benefit from away days – perhaps in a hotel at a weekend. Time is available for longer discussions of goals, plans and strategies than can occur at lunchtime team meetings. Practices have to meet the cost, which is a measure of their commitment. Staff have to give up their leisure time, sometimes unpaid. To ensure success, the away days need careful planning, structure and leadership. Outside help from an experienced facilitator is an advantage. These sessions can follow a residential multi-team workshop, and be combined with in house learning.

'In-house' team development

Teamwork involves a continuing learning process. Whatever the preliminary stages for preparing and motivating a team to learn, the team must eventually get down to work on its own real tasks and problems, with its own personnel working in context. There are several options that might apply in different settings:

- workbook only, self-resourced
- workbook plus facilitator
- facilitator only
- team development consultant only.

Some teams have had the motivation and the skill to do their own team building with the help of a workbook, such as those of Munro (1991) or Pritchard and Pritchard (1992). If this is successful, the team benefits from the confidence gained by achieving the necessary learning, and previously hidden skills in facilitation and leadership may emerge. At the end of the learning module, there is a better chance that the momentum will be maintained, either as continued team development, or merging it with management development. The ultimate goal is for the practice to become a 'learning organisation' better able to manage change and keep up-to-date, whatever is happening in the outside world.

Most teams need a helping hand to get started in unfamiliar terrain, and here a facilitator, attending the first few sessions may give the team the confidence to continue. They can help with the 'team diagnosis', and suggest ways of working that best meet the needs of each team.

If conflict is more apparent than collaboration, learning will suffer. A facilitator may be able to resolve the conflict or steer around it. If, however, the diagnostic exercise reveals severe conflict, then the services of a team development (or organisation development) consultant may be needed. The consultant would then undertake their own assessment and follow their own model of learning. Consultants who have had experience with primary health care teams are at an advantage, though the problems and cure are generic. Features that strike consultants, when they first work with primary health care teams, are the complexity of primary health care and the strong commitment and intensity of feeling that it engenders. For further consideration of conflict in teams, see Huntington (1981b) and Pritchard and Pritchard (1992).

Facilitator development

Facilitation in primary health care is a new professional activity, whose boundaries are uncertain. Surveys (for example, Bostock, 1992) have given a good idea of the nature of the role. Some excellent training exists, but facilitators mostly feel they need more. The general impression was that facilitators were doing an exacting job for which they needed more skill training. The notion that their function was as a catalyst in the development of a learning organisation was appealing to them.

In an attempt to meet some of these training needs, CAIPE and the Department of Social Science and Administration at the London School of Economics carried out a questionnaire survey, before setting up training. The respondents ranked their training needs in the following order:

1. Building effective teams
2. Management of change
3. Developing leadership skills
4. Developing facilitative and influencing skills
5. Involving patients in service development
6. Linking primary health care and other organisations and networks

There was little support for developing management skills, organisation design nor the application of information technology.

The 'learning organisation'

The 'learning organisation' is a concept that unifies many aspects of primary health care and interprofessional working and education. It may help to clarify and co-ordinate the many and diverse interests at work in this field. The idea is not new, and has common roots with the basic work on team development at MIT (Argyris and Schön, 1978). It has gained wide acceptance in industrial and public service organisations, particularly for management of change (Beckhard and Pritchard, 1992), and is now having an impact on learning in medical institutions in the UK. Primary health care, with its many strands of professional work, and its complex organisational structure, presents an ideal opportunity to apply this approach.

Team development and personal development are each a part of management development. Unless an organisation is changing to meet constantly changing circumstances, it will slip backwards. Development can be regarded as a learning cycle against a moving background, so the result is a spiral. We need to ensure that the direction of the spiral is upwards towards our goals, not downwards in the direction of chaos. Similarly, the maintenance of professional competence, clinical audit, and the implementation of health promotion, all share this model of the learning spiral. A learning organisation, made up of individuals committed to learning, can more easily take change in its stride. This can be summarised as follows:

- Bringing about change in an individual or an organisation requires *learning*, that is a change in knowledge, skills or attitudes, which is reflected in changed behaviour.
- It is *people* who learn, but their collective learning can be reflected in changes in the way their organisation functions.
- If this learning becomes a continuing process, then the organisation can be seen as a *'learning organisation'*.

The team as a 'learning organisation'

Nine features of a learning organisation are listed below (from Pritchard, W., personal communication):

1. A team must be driven by their vision of the future, not the past, (though they can learn from the past).
2. The values and the priorities of the team, and of team members, must be made explicit. Values cannot all be shared, but they need to be understood and accepted.

3. All team members must be open and prepared to innovate and acknowledge mistakes made and lessons learned.
4. 'Learning' needs to be combined with 'doing' in all the team's activities.
5. Improvement in learning must be acknowledged and rewarded, not just improvement in performance.
6. Team strategies and plans should be flexible. Planning must be seen as a learning process (for example, care plans).
7. Information needed to carry out tasks must be shared openly, and updated in response to learning by experience.
8. Training must be a catalyst for further learning and doing.
9. Becoming a learning organisation is a fundamental change, and must be managed as such.

For the learning organisation to achieve desired, but ever-changing, goals there must be a constant monitoring and tuning of the learning process. We need to keep 'learning about learning' as second nature – so-called 'double loop learning' (Argyris and Schön, 1978; Argyris, 1993).

Issues for research and development of teamwork

Team development in the UK has begun to make serious progress only in the past four years. Some outstanding issues for research and development are described below.

Public and political pressure is strong for general practice and primary health care to develop an effective, economical and user-friendly service. However, the pace of change (organisational, technological, clinical, demographic and social) is so great that it is likely to overwhelm even the most go-ahead practices. The less competent and the overtly dysfunctional practices and teams will have an even harder time, and so the gap between the teams that function best and worst is likely to widen (Pringle, 1989). Compared to other developed countries, this performance gap is already unacceptably large. So how can the range of quality and effectiveness be narrowed? Teams at the dysfunctional end of the range are likely to need more help (for example, from facilitators), help of a different kind to suit their learning needs, and possibly the judicious application of incentives and sanctions. Should a start be made at the top end, in order to raise general standards by example and diffusion of good practice, or should sights be set on the teams and practices that are finding it hard to cope?

A high priority for research will be to develop reliable methods of team diagnosis, of performance, competency and value for money over a wide range of activities. This research is under way in several centres (for example, Poulton and West, 1993; and Pearson, P. and Spencer, J., personal communication).

New information technology is proving a useful tool for handling clinical and administrative data in general practice, and making audit easier (Lawrence *et al.*, 1990). To what extent will this tool become available to other members of the PHC team? Will they share a common clinical record? Will problems of confidentiality and accountability be overcome? Will computerised decision support be able to cross professional boundaries? These issues will have to be faced if information technology is to enhance teamwork rather than create new barriers. Although reliable methods of learning to improve teamwork are available, alternatives should be explored and evaluated. For example, the Swedish method of team-building linked to organisation design (Rosenqvist *et al.*, 1990) shows great potential, and could provide some useful 'tools' for facilitators, such as conceptual and goal modelling.

Family Health Services Authorities have a new and evolving role in fostering a 'managed' PHC service, of which teamwork will be an essential ingredient. Will this be done in a way that supports or inhibits autonomous group working? Joint commissioning projects offer the opportunity for teamwork to extend more widely into community services and shared care with hospitals. The prospect that the community care manager, to be appointed under the Community Care Act (Secretary of State for Health, 1990), might be located in PHC, could result in greatly enhanced co-ordination of community care and teamwork.

The new GP contract, and fundholding in particular, are having profound effects on primary health care (both positive and negative) that are not yet clearly evaluated. 'Patients First' and the Patient's Charter are highlighting the very real difficulty of involving patients in expressing their needs, both at the one-to-one level and the organisational level. Severe conflict and misunderstanding within teams is bound to inhibit effective teamwork. Do we have the methods and the resources to restore effectiveness, if not harmony?

In conclusion

This chapter has concentrated on the practical aspects of learning to work in a team, but conflicting professional goals and values may be hard to reconcile. Is some harmonisation of goals and values a necessary or an achievable aim? Each team must plot its best path in its own unique context.

The wider use of facilitators could be a critical opportunity to bring about change. But who is their client: their employer or the team? What does the future hold for facilitators of teamwork? What do they need it terms of training and career and personal development?

As a finale, teams might ask themselves some questions, starting with the personal benefits of team working, and leading to a broader perspective of teamwork as an effective and adaptable way of providing health care.

Questions about team working

- Am I happy working in my team?
- Does it give me a feeling of fulfilment and scope for personal development?
- Is it a happy team for all its members?
- Are we a committed team?
- Are we good at adapting to change, and managing it actively?
- Is ours a learning organisation? Do we continue to learn about learning?
- **Is ours an effective team?** What criteria of effectiveness do we use? How do we know when these criteria are met?

References

Adelaide Medical Centre primary health care team (1991), 'A primary health care team manifesto', *British Medical Journal*, 41, pp. 31–3.

Allsop, J. (1990), *Changing Primary Health Care: the work of facilitators* (London: King's Fund).

Argyris, C. and Schön, D. A. (1978), *Organizational learning* (Reading, Mass: Addison-Wesley).

Argyris, C. (1983), *On organizational learning* (Cambridge, Mass: Blackwell).

Barclay report (1982), *Social workers, their role and tasks* (London: Bedford Square Press).

Beckhard, R. (1972), 'Organizational issues in team delivery of health care', *Milbank Memorial Quarterly*, 50, pp. 287–316.

Beckhard, R. and Pritchard, W. (1992), *Changing the Essence. The art of creating and leading fundamental change in organizations* (San Francisco: Jossey-Bass).

Belbin, M. (1981), *Management teams: why they succeed or fail* (Oxford: Heinemann Professional).

Bostock, Y. (1992), *Facilitator strategy review: a survey of primary care facilitators*

(Oxford: The National Facilitator Development Project, HEA Primary Health Care Unit, Churchill Hospital, Oxford OX3 7LJ).

Bruce, N. (1980), *Teamwork for Preventive Care* (Research Studies Press: Chichester: John Wiley & Sons).

CAIPE (1988), *Report on a National Survey of Interprofessional Education in Primary Health Care* (London: National Centre for the Advancement of Interprofessional Education in Primary Health and Community Care).

Cooper, L. and Hingley, P. (1988), 'Occupational stress among general practitioners', *Journal of Management in Medicine*, 3, pt 2, pp. 96–106.

Department of Health (1989) *General Practice in the National Health Service: A new contract* (London: Department of Health).

DHSS (1981), *The Primary Health Care Team*, Report of a joint working group of the Standing Medical Advisory Committee and the Standing Nursing and Midwifery Advisory Committee (London: DHSS).

DHSS (1986), *Community Nursing Review. Neighbourhood Nursing – a focus for care*, Cumberlege Report (London: HMSO).

Gilmore, M. Bruce, N. and Hunt, M. (1974), *The work of the nursing team in general practice* (London: Council for the Education and Training of Health Visitors).

Göranzon, B. (1993), *The Practical Intellect* (Berlin: Springer-Verlag).

Gregson, B., Cartlidge, A. and Bond, J. (1991), *Interprofessional Collaboration in Primary Health Care Organizations*, Occasional Paper no. 52 (London: Royal College of General Practitioners).

Hockey, L. and Buttimore, A. (1970), *Co-operation in patient care: studies of district nurses attached to hospital and general medical practices* (London: Queen's Institute of District Nursing).

Holm, H. A. and Coles, C. R. (1993), *Learning in Medicine* (Oslo: Scandinavian University Press, and Oxford University Press).

Huntington, J. (1981a) 'Time orientations in the collaboration of social workers and general practitioners', *Social Science and Medicine*, 15A, p. 203.

Huntington, J. (1981b), *Social Work and General Medical Practice: collaboration or conflict?* (London: George Allen & Unwin).

Jones, R. V. H. (1986), *Working Together – Learning Together*, Occasional paper no 33 (London: Royal College of General Practitioners).

Knight, S. and Gann, R. (1988), *A directory of self-help organizations* (London: Chapman & Hall Medical).

Lawrence, M., Coulter, A. and Jones, L. (1990), 'A total audit of preventive procedures in 45 practices caring for 430 000 patients', *British Medical Journal*, 300, pp. 1501–3.

Marsh, G. (1991), *Efficient care in general practice* (Oxford: Oxford University Press).

Munro, K. (ed.) (1991), *Teamworking in Practice. Anticipatory care in practice* (Oxford: Radcliffe Medical Press).

Poulton, B.C. and West, M. A. (1993), 'Effective multidisciplinary teamwork in primary health care', *Journal of Advanced Nursing*, 18, pp. 918–25.

Pringle, M. (1989), 'The quality divide in primary care', *British Medical Journal*, 299, p. 470.

Pritchard, P. (1981), *Manual of Primary Health Care*, 2nd edn (Oxford: Oxford University Press).

Pritchard, P. (1993), *Partnership with Patients. A practical guide to starting a patient participation group*, 3rd edn (London: Royal College of General Practitioners).

Pritchard, P., Low, K. and Whalen, M. (1984), *Management in General Practice* (Oxford: Oxford Medical Publications).

Pritchard, P. and Pritchard, J. (1992), *Developing Teamwork in Primary Health Care: a practical workbook* (Oxford: Oxford University Press). (Second edition 'Developing Teamwork in Primary and Shared Care', forthcoming 1994.)

RCGP (1985), 'What Sort of Doctor? Assessing quality of care in general practice', *Report from general practice*, 23 (London: Royal College of General Practitioners).

Rosenqvist, U., Larsson, K. and Carlson, A. (1990), 'Experiences from the Stockholm Diabetes Control Programme,' in *Treatment of Insulin-dependent Diabetes Mellitus* (National Board of Health and Welfare, Drug Information Committee, Sweden).

Rubin, I. R. and Beckhard, R. (1972), 'Factors influencing the effectiveness of health teams', *Milbank Memorial Fund Quarterly*, 50(3), 317–37.

Rubin, I. R. Plovnick, M. S. and Fry, R. E. (1975), *Improving the co-ordination of care: a program for health team development* (Harvard, Mass: Ballinger).

Secretary of State for Health (1990), *National Health Service and Community Care Act*, ch. 19, Part III, 'Community Care England and Wales' sections 42–50, pp. 50–60.

Secretary of State for Health (1992), *The Health of the Nation. A strategy for health in England*, Cm 1986 (London: HMSO).

Seebohm report (1968), *Report of the committee on Local Authority and allied Personal Social Services*, Cmnd 3703 (London: HMSO).

Spratley, J. (1989), *Disease prevention and health promotion in primary health care, Team workshops organised by the Health Education Authority* (London: HEA).

Spratley, J. (1990), *Joint planning for the development and management of disease prevention and health promotion strategies in primary health care: the HEA workshop programme for the development of Local Organising Teams* (London: HEA).

Tichy, N. M. (1977), *Organization design for primary health care: The case of the Martin Luther King Jr Health Center* (New York: Praeger).

West, M. A. (1990), 'The social psychology of innovation in groups', 'in M. A. West and J. L. Farr (eds), *Innovation and creativity at work* (Chichester: John Wiley).

Index

accountability 158
  to organisation 64
  to patient 64
age
  ethnicity 102–3, 105
  gender 102
  health 103
  housing 103–4, 105
ageism 101–2, 108
AIDS 171–2, 176
Area Child Protection Committee 114, 124, 129
attachments to general practice 193, 196
autonomy
  clinical 63, 64, 65
  doctors 166
  patients 63, 64

Balint, Dr 194
Barclay Report (1982) 24, 215
beneficence 59–60
Better Services for the Mentally Ill (1975) 145, 149
budget holders *see* fundholding practices
bureaucracy
  behaviour 37
  control 37–8
  decision-making 9–10, 20, 23; intraversion 25; welfare 25–6
  'iron cage' of 38, 39
  public 38–9
  reform 78
  self-serving 39

cancer 171–4, 176, 177–8
care managers *see* case managers
'Care Programme Approach' 148
carers *see* informal care
Caring for People (1989) 18
  locality nursing 49
  mental health services 146–7, 149–50; joint planning 151

social care 49–50
case (care) managers
  mental health services 147, 152, 153
  role 200
catchment areas and collaboration 152
'cell' systems 216
child care 111–12, 130–3
  approaches 112–13
  co-ordination 113–15
  emphasis 49
  health visitors 91
  interprofessional work 116–30
  responsibilities 50
  social workers 115–16
Child Protection Register 114, 115
  conduct of 116, 127
  enquiries to 125
Children Act (1989) 49–50, 150
  impact 100
Children Ill-treated or Neglected in their Own Homes (1950) 115
Citizen's Advice Bureau 104
Cleveland Report (1987) 116
clinical audit 45
clinical autonomy 63, 64, 65
clinical directorates 45
  importance 63
clinical management 63
clinical psychologists 142, 156
clinicians
  and contracts 82–4
  needs assessment 88
  perspective 77
  resource allocation 58–69
  role 79–81
  see also consultants; nurses
codes of conduct 57, 58
collaboration *see* interprofessional work; teamwork
College of General Practitioners (Royal) 192, 194
Colwell Report (1974) 115

233

committed teamwork 208–9
communication, interprofessional
    106, 108
    mental health services 139
community care
    definition 95
    elderly people 97, 104
    mentally ill people 137, 146–7;
        underfunding 149, 150
Community Care: Agenda for Action
    see Griffiths Report (1988)
community mental health centres
    (CMHCs) 153
community psychiatric nurses
    (CPNs) 140, 141, 142, 150, 156
community services
    definition 97
    elderly care 97
competition
    and contracts 75, 82–5
    interprofessional issues 107, 109
    introduction ,197, 198
competitive tendering 50
Confederation of Health Service
    Employees (COHSE) 43, 44
conferences, child protection 114,
    125, 129–30
confidence, professional 31
confidentiality
    child care 116
    ethical issues 60
    and interprofessional
collaboration 15
    palliative care 174, 176
consent, informed 167
consultants
    and contracts 83–4
    intraprofessional divide 48
    and managers 75, 80–1, 84
    and market 76
    and purchasers 76, 80
    teamwork 226
    see also clinicians
consumerism 21, 24
contracts
    benefits 78
    and competition 75, 82–5
    definition 72
    effects 90
    GP 197–8, 217

convenient teamwork 207–8
core group 114
Cox, Dr 166, 176
Cumberlege Report (1983) 48,
    220

Dawson Report (1920) 187
death
    attitudes to 168–71
    management of 165–8
decision-making
    bureaucratic approach 9–10, 20,
        23; intraversion 25; welfare
        25–6
    consumerism 21, 24
    democratic procedures 20, 23
    informal caring 22, 24; criticism
        26
    judicial approach 21, 24;
        criticism 26
    managerial alternative 21, 23
    managers 58–63, 65–9
    market alternative 20–1, 23
    mix 29
    palliative care 167–8
    voluntarism 22, 24
degenerative illnesses 166, 171–4,
    176
democratic decision-making 20, 23
demographic changes 96, 138
district nurses 186, 190–1
Doctors' Charter (1966) 16
double-loop learning 228

education
    of elderly people 104
    mental health services 150–1, 156
    palliative care 178–80
elderly care 95–101, 107–9
    needs 101–5
    service provision 105–7
equity 63, 66–7
    mental health services 158
essential teams 210
ethics
    definition 58–9
    issues 59–61, 64–7, 81
    palliative care 175–6
    and professionalisation 11
    resource constraints 86–7

ethnicity
    child protection 127, 131
    elderly people 102-3, 105
    mental health services 151

facilitators 220, 221-2, 225-6
fairness 63, 66-7
family care *see* informal care
Family Doctors' Charter (1966) 193
Family Health Service Authorities
    (FHSAs) 46, 221-2, 229
Family Practitioner Service 46
fundholding practices
    introduction 198
    management issues 47-8
    mental health services 156
    purchaser-provider split 72

gender differences
    child protection 131
    elderly people 102; ethnicity
        103
    management 43, 44-5
general management 43-9
general practitioners (GPs)
    child care 116, 118-20, 126-7,
        128, 132; interdisciplinary
        collaboration 128-9, 130;
        interprofessional contacts
        121-2; procedural issues
        124-5, 126
    community beds 85
    contracts 197-8, 217
    elderly care 103
    fundholding 47-8; introduction
        198; mental health services
        156; purchaser-provider split 72
    history 188-9, 192-4, 196-9
    and informal carers 104
    intraprofessional divide 48
    management 45-8
    mental health services 140-2,
        155-6, 157-8
    palliative care 177
    referrals 76
Green Paper (1968) 13, 16-17
Green Paper (1970) 17
Grey Book (1972) 41
Griffiths Report (1983) 23, 40-1,
    42

Griffiths Report (1988) 18, 45,
    199-200
    mental health services 146, 149-50

health centres 193-4
    Dawson Report (1920) 187
Health Education Authority (HEA)
    218-20
Health Maintenance Organisations
    (HMOs) 47
Health Services and Public Health
    Act (1968) 16
health visitors
    child care 116, 118, 119-20, 127;
        constraints on interprofessional
        work 123, 124;
        interdisciplinary collaboration
        129, 130; interprofessional
        contacts 121, 122; procedural
        issues 124, 126; training 121
    history 186, 188, 191-2, 193
    mental health services 141
home care teams 176-8
homeless people 159
hospices 177-6
Hospital Plan (1962) 144
housing, elderly people 103-4, 105

income, elderly people 104
indicative prescribing 47
individualism
    and attitudes to death 169-70
    and utilitarianism 59-61
informal care 22, 24
    criticism 26
    of elderly people 96, 102, 104;
        ethnicity 103
    of mentally ill people 139-40
    palliative care 172, 178;
        hospices 174
information technology 229
informed consent 167
Interdisciplinary Child Protection
    Conference 114, 125-6, 129-30
interorganisational relations, child
    protection
    exchange 112
    mandated co-ordination 112-15,
        122
    power/resource dependency 112

interprofessional work 9–10, 30–2
  child protection: consensus
    128–30; constraints 122–4;
    contacts 121–2; co-operation
    111, 116, 118; co-ordination
    111, 112–15; empirical study
    116–21
  communication 106, 108
  Family Doctors' Charter 193
  mental health: improvement
    150–3; necessity 138–9;
    primary care 155–9; reasons
    142–50; unmet need 139–41
  relationships 48
  see also teamwork
intraprofessional divide 48
intraprofessional relationships 48
  Family Doctors' Charter 193

jargon, professional 106, 108
joint planning, mental health
    services 151–2
judicial approach to
    decision-making 21, 24
  criticism 26
just desserts, ethics of 60–1

key workers
  child protection 114
  mental health services 140, 148,
    152–3
knowledge mix 30–1

language, interprofessional 106, 108
lawyers 119, 121
learning organisations 227–8
Local Organising Teams (LOTs)
    218–20
loyalty, professional 33

'Making a Reality of Community
    Care' (1986) 145–6
managed markets 106–7
management
  clinical 63
  general 43–9
managerial alternative 21, 23
managers
  case 147, 152, 153
  and consultants 75, 80–1, 84

and contracts 73–4, 83, 84, 90
  decision-making 58–63, 65–9
  needs assessment 84, 88–9
  role 75–6, 77–9
  teamwork 221–3
  views of 57
manifestos, team 220–1
Maria Colwell Report (1974) 115
markets
  and consultants 76
  and decision-making 20–1, 23
  definition 73
  managed 106–7
  and public services 73–5
Medical Officers of Health 188,
    189–90, 193
men, elderly 102
  ethnicity 103
Mental Health Act (1959) 143,
    144
Mental Health Act (1983) 24, 143,
    145
mental health services 137–8,
    159–60
  interprofessional collaboration
    138–53; structural issues 153–9
mental illness
  definition 138
  extent 137–8
Mental Treatment Act (1930) 143
midwives 90–1
morale
  elderly care 108
  general practitioners 188
multidisciplinary assessments 96,
    100, 105–6
multiprofessional work 10
mutual respect 64, 68, 101, 102

National Assistance Act (1948)
    143–4
National Health Service and
    Community Care Act (1990)
    10, 45, 200
  elderly care 96, 101, 104, 108
National Society for the Prevention
    of Cruelty to Children (NSPCC)
    114, 116
National Union of Public
    Employees (NUPE) 43

needs assessment 78, 87–9
  elderly care 96–7, 101–5, 107
  managers 85, 88–9
  mentally ill people 148
  and purchasers 76, 80
Nightingale, Florence 40–1, 42,
  43, 44
nominal teamwork 207, 208
non-malevolence 65–6
nurses
  changing role 49, 50
  child care 119, 121
  community beds 85
  community psychiatric (CPNs)
    140, 141, 142, 150, 156
  and contracts 82–3
  elderly care 98–9
  general management 42–4
  see also clinicians

organisational-oriented 'full' teams
  213

paediatricians 118–19, 127, 128,
  132, 133
  Cleveland affair 116
  constraints on interprofessional
    work 123
  experience 120
  interprofessional contacts 122
  procedural issues 124, 125
palliative care 165–72, 181
  education implications 173–80
  hospices and multidisciplinary
    approaches 177–6
  hospital–home interface 176–8
paternalism 64, 90, 179
patient-centred 'intrinsic' teams
  212
Pink, Graham 168, 180
point of authorisation 62
point of legitimisation 61
point of satisfaction 62
police and child protection 116,
  118–19, 127, 128, 132
  experience 120, 121
  constraints on interprofessional
    work 123
  interprofessional contacts 121,
    122

practice managers 48
prescribing, indicative 47
primacy 65
primary health care 185–200
  definition 186
  teams 213–14; mental health
    services 155–9; palliative care
    177–8
prime responsibility 65, 68
private sector
  changing role 50
  elderly care 96, 98–9, 100
process-orientated teamwork 214
professional frameworks
  differences 96, 98–100
  nurses 98–9
  private sector 96, 98–9, 100
  social services 95, 98–100
  voluntary sector 96, 98–9, 100
professionals
  characteristics 39
  codes of conduct 57, 58
  definition 57
  and managers 57–8
  resource allocation 58–69
  restrictive practices 39–40
  and semi-professionals 40
professions
  conflicts: with each other 14–18;
    with policy-makers 18–19;
    with theorists 12–14
  professionalisation 11–12
  and welfare 27–8
providers
  and contracts 82
  definition 72
  risks of services 101
  role 72, 86
  see also purchaser–provider split
psychiatrists 156
  child care 119
  community psychiatric nurses
    (CPNs) 140, 141, 142, 150, 156
psychiatry
  changing role 145
  joint planning 152
  sectorisation 152
  stature 143
  and unmet need 139
psychologists, clinical 142, 156

purchaser–provider split
  bureaucracy 9
  introduction 46, 50
  policy-makers 18
  public service bureaucracies 33
  roles 72
purchasers
  and clinicians 76, 80
  contracts 84, 90
  definition 72
  needs assessment 87–9
  and public health 76–7
  role 86

Resource Allocation Working Party
  (RAWP) 45
respect, mutual 64, 68, 101, 102
respite care 173
Royal College of General
  Practitioners 192, 194
Royal College of Nursing (RCN) 42, 43
Royal Commission on the NHS
  (1979) 14, 17–18

Salmon Report (1966) 41, 42
sectorisation and collaboration 152
Seebohm Report (1968) 17, 23,
  145, 195, 214
self-reports, child abuse 112
senile dementia 138
service agreements *see* contracts
service delivery units 76, 86
skill mix 29–30
social services
  elderly care 95, 98–100
  and informal carers 104
social workers
  child care 118, 119, 127, 128,
  132–3; constraints on
  interprofessional work 123,
  124; experience 120, 121;
  interdisciplinary collaboration
  129, 130; interprofessional
  contacts 121, 122; procedural
  issues 124–5, 126
  role 114, 115–16
  history 186, 191–2, 194–5, 196
  mental health services 140, 142,
  154, 156, 157–8
  Seebohm Report 145, 195

task-orientated 'full' teams
  212–13, 214
teachers and child protection 116,
  118–20, 126, 127, 128
  interdisciplinary collaboration
  130
  interprofessional contacts 121,
  122
  training 121
teams
  in changing environment 216
  co-operation 207, 208
  definition 206–7
  diagnosis 209–10
  as learning organisation 227–8
  organisation-orientated/full 213
  patient-centred/intrinsic/
  essential 212
  primary health care 213–14;
  mental health services 155–9;
  palliative care 176–7
  size 215–16
  task-orientated/functional 212–13
  time dimension 216–17
teamwork
  benefits 210–12
  committed 208–9
  convenient 207–8
  Health Education Authority
  218–20
  nominal 207, 208
  prevention and health promotion
  217–18
  task/process orientated 214
  see also interprofessional work
terminal care *see* palliative care
Terminal Care Support Team 177
training
  child protection work 120–1,
  125–6, 128
  mental health services 150–1
  teamwork 223; away days 225;
  basic/postbasic interdisciplinary
  223–4; in-house 225–6;
  residential workshops 224–5

underfunding
  mental health services 149–50
  resource allocation 86, 87
unitary fallacy 18

utilitarian principles
  definition 59
  limitation 59
utilitarianism 91
  and individualism 59–61

voluntary sector
  changing role 50
  decision-making 22, 24
  elderly care 104, 107;
    professional framework 96,
    98–9, 100

whistleblowing 63, 66–7, 168, 180
women
  elderly 102; ethnicity 103
  and management 43, 44–5
Working for Patients (1989) 18, 45,
    47
  locality nursing 49
Working Together 114
workload figures 82, 84, 86

Younghusband, Dame Eileen
    194–5